TAI CHI FOR

SENIORS OVER 60

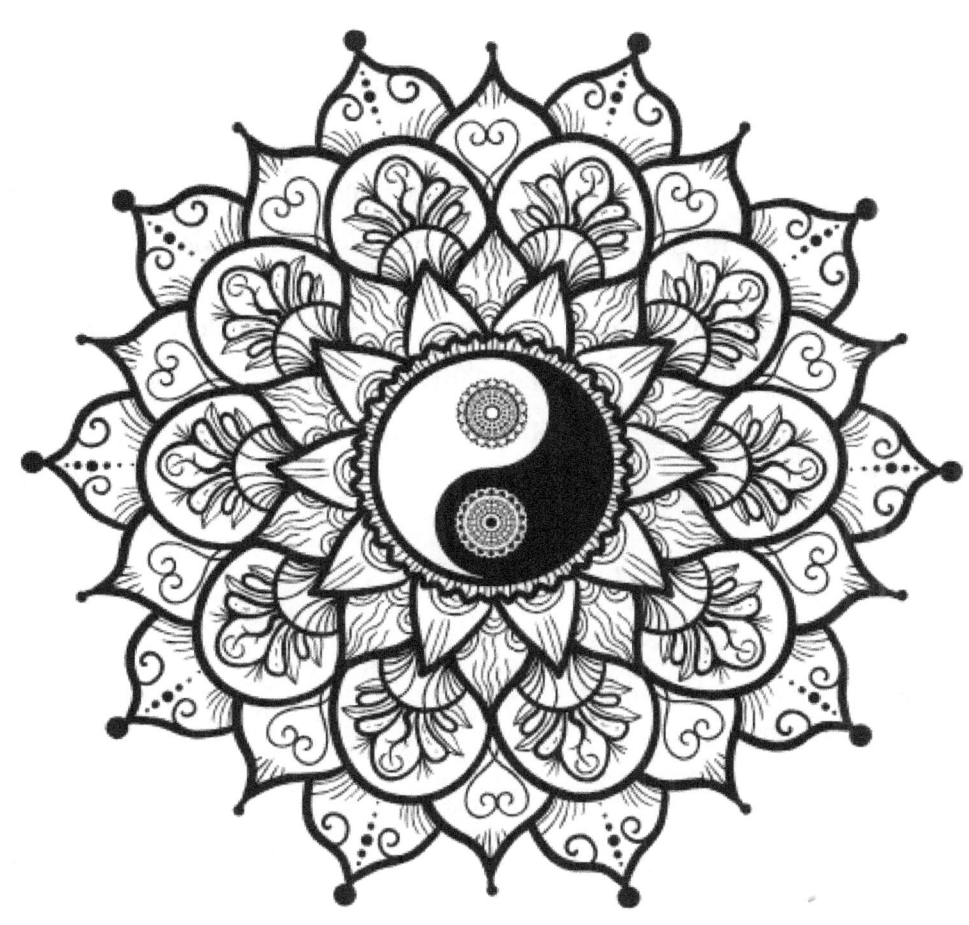

Copyright Notice

© 2025. All Rights Reserved.

No part of this publication may be reproduced, distributed, or transmitted in any form or by any means, including photocopying, recording, or other electronic or mechanical methods, without the prior written permission of the publisher, except in the case of brief quotations embodied in critical reviews and certain other non-commercial uses permitted by copyright law.

Disclaimer

This book is designed to provide educational information on the topic of Tai Chi. It is sold with the understanding that the publisher and author are not engaged in rendering medical, health, or any other kind of personal professional advice. The reader should consult a qualified medical professional before beginning any new exercise program, including the one described in this book.

By undertaking the exercises and techniques in this book, you assume all risks associated with them. The author and publisher shall have neither liability nor responsibility to any person or entity with respect to any loss or damage caused, or alleged to have been caused, directly or indirectly, by the information contained in this book.

ISBN: 979-8-234-00344-7
Cover & interior design: Fabiana Renacer
Published by: Fabiana Renacer
Printed in the United States of America

For every soul who proves that age is no match for strength,
grace, and transformation.
May every gentle movement in this book guide you
toward renewed health, lasting energy,
and the simple joy of living life to the fullest.

It begins with finding stillness in the body
to create balance in the mind.
And from that quiet space... graceful movement blossoms.

FABIANA RENACER

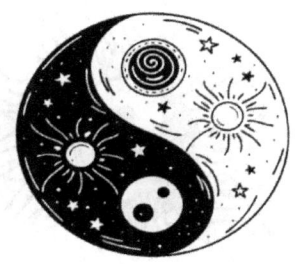

DEDICATION

To the wise soul who understands that aging is not a loss, but a gentle unfolding—a new landscape you are meant to explore with grace, curiosity, and an open heart. This book is dedicated to you, who has ever heard the whisper—or the shout—that with age comes limitation. Consider this my gentle, powerful, and deeply human response to that voice. A reminder that your story is still being written, one breath, one movement, one mindful moment at a time.

It is for you, who chooses to greet each day not with resignation, but with presence. For you, who decides to move not with fear, but with curiosity—and to speak to your body not with criticism, but with the compassion it has always deserved. It is for you, who knows that the deepest strength is often found in softness, and that true balance begins not just in the body, but in a peaceful mind and a willing spirit.

And if you have ever stood before the mirror and wondered, "Has my time for new beginnings passed?"—I offer you these pages as a testament to a beautiful truth: Your time is not behind you. It is here. It is now. In this moment. In this breath. In this gentle movement. This is where your new story begins — not as a chapter of decline, but as an era of your own rediscovery, resilience, and quiet power. This book is more than a guide. I created it to be your companion. It reflects my belief in you—a belief I hold with unwavering certainty, rooted in the knowledge that you are capable of more than you have been led to believe.

Yes, you can.

You really, truly can.

And I am honored to walk this path with you.

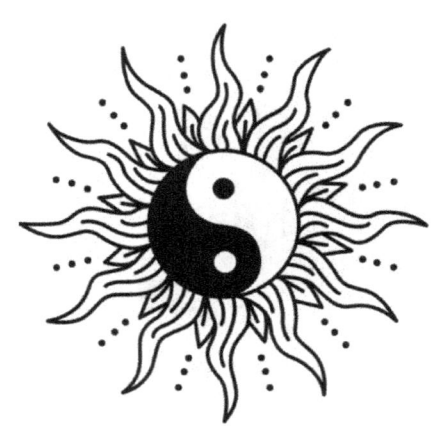

ACKNOWLEDGMENTS

My deepest gratitude first to God—the source of my strength, my clarity, and my peace. This project was nurtured in silence and prayer, and it was His guidance that gently led me through every step.

To my husband, whose quiet courage and steady love have been my anchor. You stood by me not with grand gestures, but with a presence that made everything feel possible.

To my sons, now men walking their own beautiful paths across the world: you are my reason and my inspiration. In many ways, this book was born from the space between us—a mother's loving attempt to keep moving forward with purpose, until the day our paths bring us together again.

To my mother, whose belief in me has never wavered. Your faith has been a quiet echo in my heart, reminding me to keep going even when the way felt unclear.

To my family, my friends, and the quiet supporters who encouraged me to share this message with the world—thank you for reminding me that healing, growth, and contribution do not come with an expiration date.

And finally, to you, the reader: thank you for trusting these pages. Your presence here is more than a gesture—it is a quiet act of courage, a choice to honor yourself in ways that truly matter. It is my sincere hope that as you move through this program, you feel deeply supported, genuinely respected, and gently awakened to all that is still possible within you.

Tai Chi, in the end, is more than movement. It is a homecoming—a return to balance, to breath, to trust in your own rhythm. No matter where you begin, or how far you feel you've come, your body is always, always inviting you back home.

PROLOGUE

You might be opening this book with a quiet hope tucked inside—
the hope of moving with ease again, of feeling steadier on your feet,
or simply of reconnecting with a part of yourself that life's pace has pushed aside.
Maybe your body feels stiffer than it once did, or balance asks for more attention.
Perhaps you've wondered whether it's "too late" to begin something new.
If so, I want you to know this from the very first page: **you are not behind, and you are not alone.**
I did not arrive at Tai Chi through tradition, but through a lifelong search for practices that make life gentler, clearer, and more meaningful.

My background in yoga, mindful breathing, and emotional coaching opened many doors—
but Tai Chi opened a deeper one.
I discovered movements that were soft yet powerful, slow yet intelligent, simple yet transformative.
And I saw how people—especially in this stage of life—
began to move not only with more stability, but with more dignity, confidence, and calm.

Over the years, I witnessed small miracles:
a step that no longer felt uncertain,
a back that released its long-held tension,
a breath that arrived deeper and kinder.
Eyes brightened. Shoulders opened.
People rediscovered the joy of moving without fear.

This book was created from those moments.
It is a **safe, progressive, real-life program** made for adults who want to feel better in their bodies—
without strain, without pressure, and without the unrealistic demands of traditional fitness.
You don't need experience, flexibility, or perfect posture.
All you need is a few minutes a day, a chair if needed, and a willingness to meet your body where it is, with kindness.

These 28 days are not a test.
They are an invitation.
A gentle path back to balance, strength, and inner peace—
one breath at a time.

Thank you for trusting me to accompany you.
I'm honored to walk this journey with you.

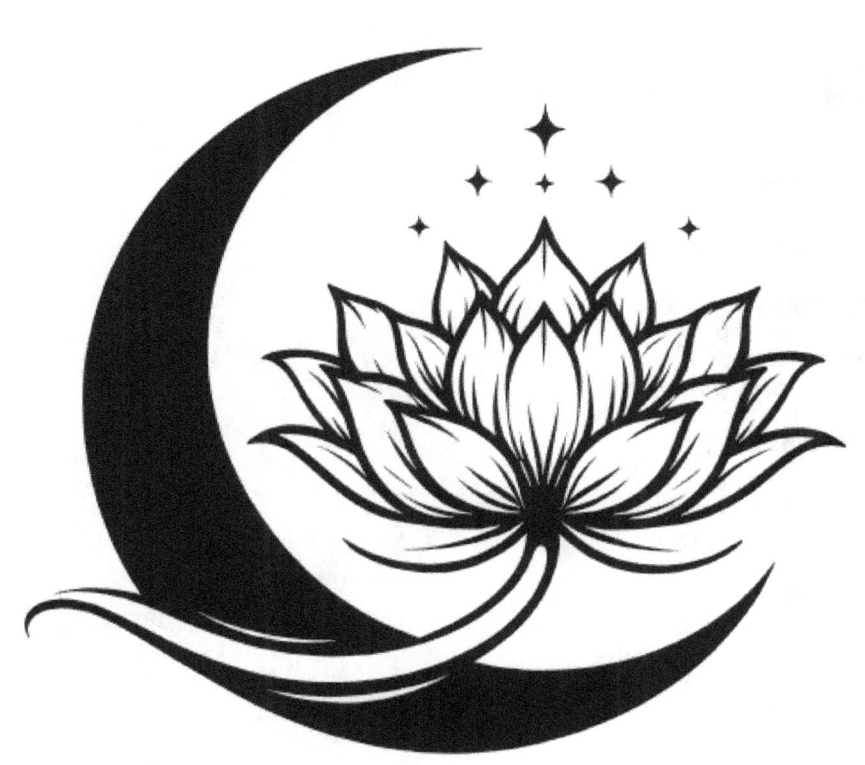

TABLE OF CONTENTS

INTRODUCTION — 1
Tai Chi today
The art of inteligent movement after 60

CHAPTER 1 — 3
Essential fundamentals to start with security and confidence

CHAPTER 2 — 5
How this 28-day program works and make it your trip

CHAPTER 3- WEEK 1- Reconnect — 7
Day 1- The tree that sends roots
Day 2- The mountain pose — 9
Day 3- Brushing the clouds — 11
Day 4- Flowing Silk — 13
Day 5- Gentle knee bend — 15
Day 6- Opening the heart — 17
Day 7- The silence that heals — 19

CHAPTER 4-WEEK 2- Strengthen — 23
Day 8- The pilar of strength
Day 9- The power beneath the surface — 25
Day 10- The core that carries you — 27
Day 11- The hips that hold you — 29
Day 12- The power of your step — 31
Day 13- The strength that bends — 33
Day 14- The to stay, the readiness to shift — 35

CHAPTER 5- WEEK 3- Expand — 37
Day 15- The to stay, the readiness to shift
Day 16- The center that moves with you — 41
Day 17- The bridge between points — 43
Day 18- The weight that's light — 45
Day 19- The balance beneath you — 47
Day 20- The spiral that holds center — 49
Day 21- The quiet center, the moving edge — 51

CHAPTER 6- WEEK 4- Flow — 53
Day 22- The stream of movement
Day 23- The wave of continuity — 57
Day 24- The river of rhythm — 59
Day 25- The circle of breath and movement — 61
Day 26- The breath that carries motion — 63
Day 27- The full current within — 65
Day 28- The flow that carries forever — 67

CHAPTER 7-Tai Chi for Memory Mood & Emotional Well-Being — 73

CHAPTER 8- Adaptations for common conditions — 76

CHAPTER 9-What Happens After the 28 Days? Your Path Forward. — 78

APPENDIX & RESOURCES — 81

INTRODUCTION
Tai Chi today
The art of Intelligent movement after 60

What Is Tai Chi and Why Practice It After 60?

As the years pass, it's natural to feel more cautious with your body.
Concerns about balance, stiffness, or injuries may appear—and they are valid.
But there is also another possibility:

What if there were a way of moving that doesn't force your body but supports it?
A practice that loosens tension, strengthens gently, and restores balance by listening to your breath.
That practice is **Tai Chi**—and this book brings it to you in a clear, safe, and accessible way.

Tai Chi: Art, Medicine, and a Gentle Path Forward

Born in ancient China, Tai Chi is not just slow movement.
It is a mind–body practice that teaches your system to move with ease instead of resistance.
Its softness is its power:
moving slowly retrains muscles, joints, and the nervous system in a safe, intelligent way.
Circular motions reduce stiffness, rooted postures improve stability, and fluid transitions teach adaptability.
Over time, this becomes a new way of inhabiting your body—with more confidence, clarity, and grace.

Why Tai Chi Speaks to You After 60

After 60, the body responds best to movement that is **smart, gentle, and consistent**—not forceful.
Modern research from Harvard, Mayo Clinic and Stanford confirms that Tai Chi can:

- Improve balance and reduce the risk of falls
- Strengthen legs and core **without impact**
- Calm stress and support deeper, easier breathing
- Improve focus, memory, and attention
- Renew vitality by improving circulation and oxygen flow

You don't need to be flexible, strong, or experienced. Tai Chi adapts to your real body, right now.

Three Adaptive Levels — Your Practice, Your Way
Every day in this 28-day journey offers three options, so you can choose what your body needs:

Level 1 – Seated Foundation
Maximum safety and clarity.
Ideal for low-energy days or when you want to focus on breath and gentle mobility.

Level 2 – Standing with Support
A safe challenge for balance, walking strength, and stability.
A chair or wall is always within reach.

Level 3 – Flowing Standing Practice
For days when you feel ready to move with more rhythm and coordination—always within a comfortable range.

These levels aren't steps to "complete"—they're choices.
You may switch between them freely. That flexibility is part of the practice.

What Tai Chi Is Not — Clearing Common Myths

- **"It's too slow to be exercise."**
Slow movement trains deep strength, stability, and joint health.

- **"I won't remember the movements."**
This program repeats simple patterns that gradually evolve. No choreography required.

- **"It's spiritual or esoteric."**
Here, Tai Chi is presented as a practical wellness practice. You choose its personal meaning.

Your Wellness Toolbox for the 28-Day Journey
To support your progress, this program includes:

- Guided videos for all three levels
- Short pauses for anxiety or better sleep
- Music suggestions to relax or energize
- An Inner Journey Notebook to track your reflections
- One-minute "micro-practices" for daily life
- Partner or group options
- A quick guide for safe movements on days of pain or fatigue

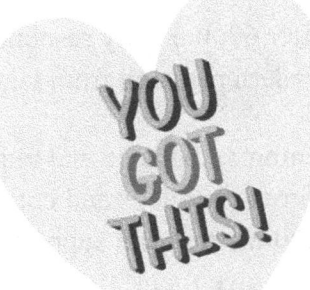

This is not a technical manual—it's a clear, compassionate companion designed to help you move with confidence

CHAPTER 1

Essential fundamentals to start with security and confidence

YOUR THREE INTERNAL PILLARS
These are your allies. You don't have to learn them: they already live within you.

1. Breath — Your Anchor

- Slow exhale = "You are safe."
- Reduces tension, supports calm movement.
- Connects mind and body so movement feels easier.

2. Balance — Your Dialogue With the Ground

- Balance can be retrained at any age.
- Slow movement teaches ankles, knees, hips to respond wisely.
- A wobble is not failure—it's practice.

3. Energy (Qi) — The Feeling of Being Aliv

- Qi is simply your body's vitality.
- Slow, continuous movement frees stiffness.
- You feel lighter, clearer, and quietly strong

POSTURE & MOVEMENT — THE STRING AND THE TREE	
IMAGE	WHAT IT MEANS
The Suspended String	A gentle lift from the crown. Shoulders soften. Alert and relaxed—not rigid.
The Rooted Tree	Feet or sitting bones grounded. Movement starts from the center, like branches supported by strong roots.

YOUR PRACTICE, YOUR RULES — THE CHAIR AS AN ALLY	
OPTION	WHY IT MATTERS
Seated Practice	Full mental and respiratory benefits, zero risk. Ideal on low-energy days.
Standing With Support	Builds balance safely with something nearby to hold.
Standing Free	A natural progression when your body feels ready.

SAFETY FIRST — THE BODY AS HOME

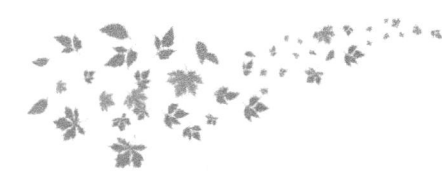

Short principles to protect joints and improve confidence:

1. **"Live Knees, Never Locked."**
   Keep a soft bend for safer balance.
2. **"Turn With Your Roots."**
   Feet and hips join the movement—no isolated twisting.
3. **"Listening Feet."**
   Notice where your weight is before moving.
4. **"The Breath Leads."**
   If tense or breathless: pause, soften, reset.

Practicing this way builds strength that lasts.

A SIMPLE BEGINNING PRACTICE

Try this before starting your 28 days.
1. Breathe
Inhale 4 counts, exhale 6 counts (×3).
2. Feel
Notice the contact of feet or sitting bones with support.
3. Listen
Soften any area asking for space—shoulders, jaw, back.
This is Tai Chi: breath, awareness, kindness.

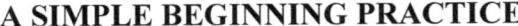

A CONCLUSION TO BEGIN

Return to this chapter whenever you need to reconnect.

The goal is not a perfect posture.
The real achievement is remembering the calm, strength and presence already inside you—waiting to be awakened.

CHAPTER 2
How this 28-day program works and make it your trip

This is not a book to leave on a shelf. It's meant to stay close: open on a table, with notes in the margins and maybe a few pages softened by use. Think of it as a travel companion, not a manual.
For the next 28 days, you're not running a race. There is no finish-line podium.
The "prize" is you: feeling more connected, safer in your steps, and calmer in your mind.
In this chapter, you'll see **how the journey is organized** and **how to adapt it** so it fits your real life—energy levels, mood, and schedule included.

YOUR JOURNEY MAP — 4 WEEKS, ONE GENTLE PROGRESSION		
WEEK	**THEME**	**WHAT YOU DEVELOP**
RECONNECT	Breathe, slow down, feel your body again.	Foundation, calm, awareness.
STRENGTHEN	Legs, core, posture.	Stability, safety, confidence.
EXPAND	Space, mobility, coordination.	Openness, rhythm, ease.
FLOW	Continuity and whole-body movement.	Integration, fluidity, natura balance.

You may repeat or linger in any week.
This program is a guide, not a rule.

A TYPICAL DAY — YOUR 10-MINUTE ROUTINE	
SECTION	**PURPOSE**
Preparation	Arrive, breathe, feel your base.
Main Movement (3 Levels)	Choose seated, supported standing, or flowing standing.
Cool-Down & Integration	Settle the nervous system and "save" the benefits.
Daily Affirmation	A phrase to carry with you during the day.
Know More	A simple insight about breath, balance, or movement.
Inner Journey Prompt	One or two reflection questions.

Practice morning, midday, or evening—whenever life allows.
Consistency beats perfection.

THE THREE LEVELS — ONE PROGRAM, MANY DOORS		
LEVEL	**HOW IT FEELS**	**WHEN TO USE IT**
Essential (Seated)	Gentle, grounding.	Tired days, beginners, pain, or recovery.
Standing with Support	Stable with challenge.	To build balance and strength safely.
Flowing Version	Continuous and soft.	Days with more energy or curiosity.

You can mix levels freely.
Listening to your body **is** the practice.

WHEN LIFE HAPPENS

Missing a day is normal.
You can: Continue with the next day, **or**
Repeat the last day, **or**
Do a **5-minute mini-practice** (Preparation + Level 1 + Cool-Down).

A thin thread of practice is stronger than long breaks of effort.

YOUR INNER JOURNEY NOTEBOOK

Use it as a quiet check-in:

- "I felt softer today."
- "My wobble didn't scare me."
- "I slept better after Day 7."
These notes reveal emotional and physical progress that the mirror cannot show.

FINAL MESSAGE — YOU HAVE THE MAP

Now you know:

- How the 4 weeks unfold
- What each day contains
- How to choose your level
- What to do when life interrupts
- How to use your Notebook and bonuses

Your journey begins next: **Week 1 — Reconnect**
A gentle return to your body.

I'm honored to walk these 28 days with you.

CHAPTER 3 -WEEK 1-Reconnect
Day 1- The tree that sends roots

根气息

Traditional Name: *Gen Qi Xi* — "Rooted Breathing"
Focus: To quiet your mind, reconnect with your vital center, and build a calm, stable foundation from deep stilling

> **PREPARATION (Standing or Seated)**
> • Place your feet hip width apart or sit tall with both feet grounded.
> • Allow your shoulders to drop—let the tension melt a little.
> • Soften your face, eyebrows, and jaw.
> • Inhale for 4… Exhale for 6…
> • Imagine gentle roots growing from your feet or spine into the earth.

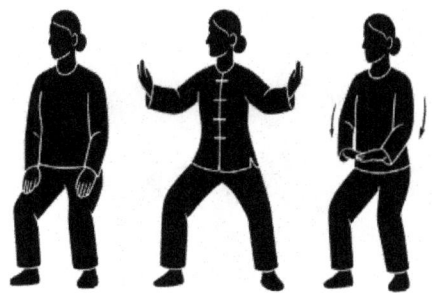

1-The Awakening Sprout

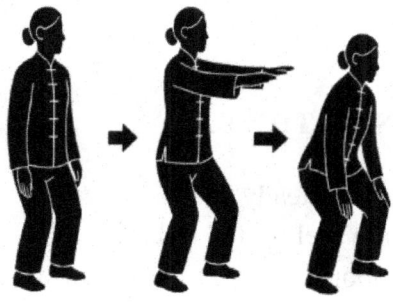

2-The Growing Tree

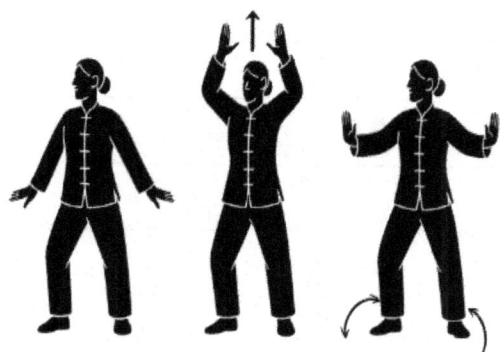

3-The Tree in the Breeze
(Subtle Sway)

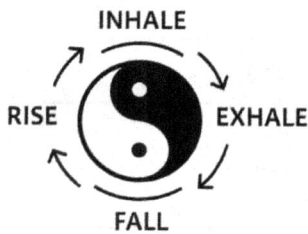

BREATHING CYCLE
INHALE
RISE — EXHALE
FALL

LEVEL 1- Awakening Sprout	LEVEL 2- Growing Tree	LEVEL 3- Tree in the Breeze
Inhale: raise both arms slowly to chest height. **Exhale:** lower them gently while keeping knees soft and feet grounded. **Repeat** 6-8 cycles with steady breathing.	**Inhale:** lift arms sideways and slightly upward. **Exhale:** lower arms slowly forming a circular path downward. Maintain upright posture and smooth coordination with breath.	**Inhale:** expand chest, feel the spine lengthen upward. **Exhale:** allow a gentle sway from ankles, returning to center. Keep balance and repeat 8-10 cycles withing comfort range.

BODY & WELLBEING BENEFITS

AREA	THERAPEUTIC EFFECT	DAILY EFFECT
Legs & Ankles	Gentle root strength	More stability- Fewer stumble
Nervous System	Softer tension- Calmer breath.	Better sleep- Less stress
Mind	Sense of precense	Feeling safer in your body

THERAPEUTIC TIPS

- Keep your eyes on a soft point in front of you.
- Move as slowly as your breath invites you.
- Seated practice is always a valid option.

REFLECTION OF THE DAY

- Where do I feel unsteady?
- What helped me feel rooted today?
- What does support mean to me right now?

JOURNAL — My Notes

_____   _____
_____   _____
_____   _____
_____   _____
_____   _____
_____   _____
_____   _____
_____   _____

DAY 2
The mountain pose

无极桩

Traditional Name: *Wu Ji Zhuang* — "The Posture of Limitless Potential"
Focus: To cultivate deep, tranquil stability. Root your body into the earth while your spine rises with quiet dignity.

> **PREPARATION & BREATHING BASE (Standing or seated)**
> ▸ Stand tall with feet hip-width apart, knees soft.
> ▸ Lengthen your spine, crown toward the sky.
> ▸ Relax shoulders and jaw; arms rest by your sides.
> ▸ Inhale for 4 counts — Exhale for 6 counts, steady and smooth.
> ▸ Feel your feet grounded, your breath anchoring your posture. The body is firm but never rigid.

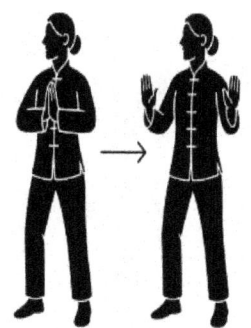

1-Tranquil Mountain (Hands at Heart)

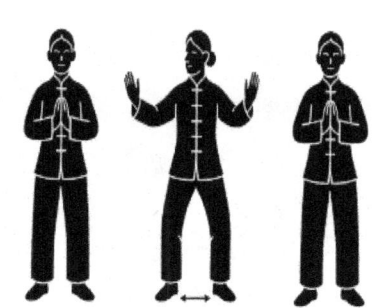

2-The Expanding Mountain

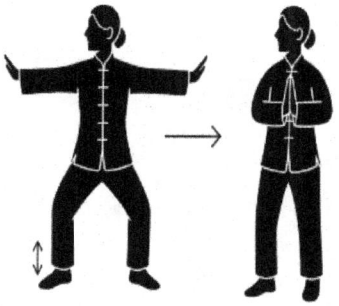

3-Mountain in the Breeze (Lateral Sway)

LEVEL 1- Tranquil Mountain
Inhale: Slowly raise your arms forward to chest height.
Exhale: Lower them softly, letting your weight root downward.
Repeat 6–8 cycles, moving with calm rhythm.

LEVEL 2- Expanding Mountain
Inhale: Lift both arms to the sides and slightly upward.
Exhale: Let them form an open circle downward to your sides.
Keep your spine tall, knees relaxed, and breath guiding movement.

LEVEL 3- Mountain in the Breeze
Begin tall, arms resting naturally.
Inhale: Expand your chest and lengthen your spine.
Exhale: Allow a gentle sway from your ankles, like wind moving softly around you.

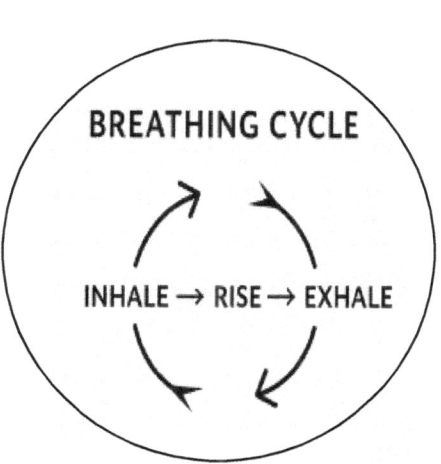

BODY & WELLBEING BENEFITS

AREA	THERAPEUTIC EFFECT	DAILY RESULT
Feet-Legs	Strengthens ankles, improves . Balance	More confidence and stability while walking
Back-Spine	Releases tension and supports alignment	Less back pain, easier upright posture
Lungs-Heart	Expands breathing capacity	Calmer pulse, greater mental clarity
Mind	Cultivates inner stillness	Reduces anxiety and improves focus

THERAPEUTIC TIPS
- Keep your gaze soft, slightly ahead of you.
- Let your breath lead the rhythm of movement.
- If you feel tired, reduce the range — calmness is more important than effort.
- Standing still is a practice of awareness — your balance is alive within quietness.

REFLECTION OF THE DAY

- What part of me feels grounded and strong today?
- When do I lose my center — physically or emotionally?
- How can I bring this sense of mountain calm into my daily life?

JOURNAL — My Notes

DAY 3
Brushing the clouds

云手

Traditional Name: *Yun Shou* — "Cloud Hands"
Focus: To release the weight in your shoulders and neck, create space for fuller breathing, and invite lightness and flow into your upper body.

PREPARATION & BASE BREATHING
Stand with feet hip-width apart or sit tall with feet grounded.
Let your shoulders melt away from your ears.
Inhale gently through the nose for 4 counts, exhale through the mouth for 6.
Imagine light clouds drifting above your shoulders — your arms follow their rhythm.

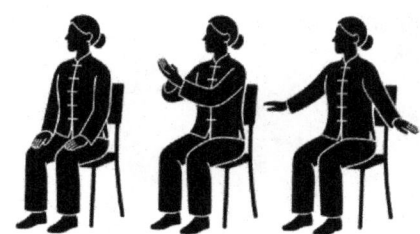

1-The Resting Cloud (Seated or Standing)

LEVEL 1 — The Resting Cloud (Seated or Standing)
Inhale: Raise both forearms in front of the chest, palms facing upward.
Exhale: Turn palms downward, lowering arms softly to the sides.
Focus: Keep shoulders relaxed, wrists fluid. Repeat 6–8 slow cycles.

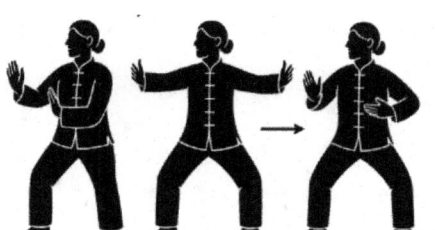

2-The Dancing Clouds

LEVEL 2 — The Dancing Clouds (Standing Flow)
Inhale: Lift arms forward to chest height, elbows relaxed.
Exhale: Open arms outward in a wide circular motion, then return to center.
Focus: Maintain upright posture and gentle knee flexion. 8–10 cycles.

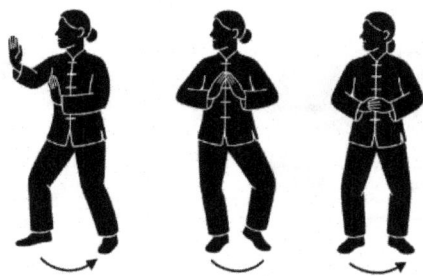

3-The Wind Moves the Clouds (Side Step)

LEVEL 3 — The Wind Moves the Clouds (Sidestep)
Inhale: Shift weight onto one foot while lifting arms outward.
Exhale: Return to center, lowering arms and alternating sides.
Focus: Feel smooth lateral weight transfer. 8–10 alternating reps.

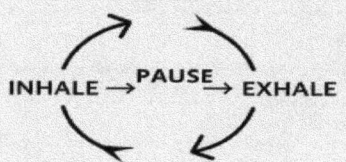

BREATHING CYCLE
INHALE → PAUSE → EXHALE

BODY & WELLBEING BENEFITS

AREA	BODY BENEFIT	DAILY EFFECT
Shoulders & Neck	Loosens chronic tension	Improves posture and mobility
Upper Back & Chest	Expands breath capacity	Reduces fatigue, improves oxigen flow
Balance & Coordination	Gentle lateral weight shifts	Enhances proprioception and fall prevention

> **THERAPEUTIC TIPS**
> Keep your eyes softly focused ahead, as if watching slow-moving clouds.
> Move your arms like silk threads — smooth, not forced.
> Breathe evenly, matching the rhythm of your movement.

REFLECTION OF THE DAY

- What tension began to release as I moved today?
- Did my breath feel lighter or more open?
- Where do I still hold tightness, I can soften next time

JOURNAL — My Notes

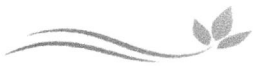

DAY 4
Flowing Silk

云手流韵

Traditional Name: *Yún Shǒu Liú Yùn* — "Flowing Silk Hands"

Focus: To synchronize breath and gentle circular motion, improving shoulder mobility and cultivating inner calm through continuous flow.

PREPARATION & BASE BREATHING

Stand (or sit) with feet hip-width apart, knees relaxed.

Breathe deeply three times: inhale to lift your spine, exhale to soften your shoulders.

Rotate wrists in slow circles, as if tracing smooth silk threads in the air.

Inhale as arms rise; exhale as they lower — 4 to 5 times with fluid continuity.

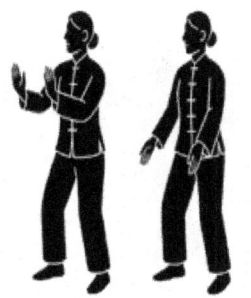

1-The Resting Cloud

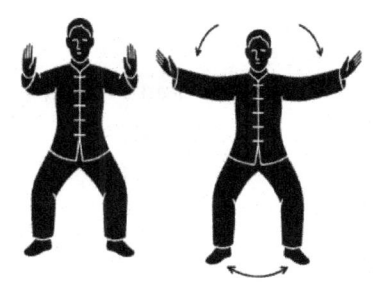

2-The Resting Cloud

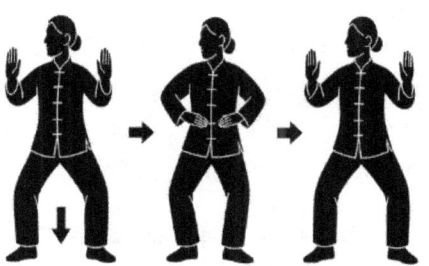

3-The Dancing Clouds

LEVEL 1 — Floating Silk (Seated or Standing)

Inhale: Lift arms to chest level, palms facing each other.

Exhale: Circle hands outward and down, smoothing cloth.

Focus: Gentle, even rhythm. 6–8 cycles.

LEVEL 2 — Weaving the Air (Standing)

Inhale: Raise both arms in a curved path upward.

Exhale: Sweep arms outward and down, tracing an infinity path.

Focus: Fluid motion through shoulders and spine. 8–10 cycles.

LEVEL 3 — Gliding Silk with Side Flow

Inhale: Shift weight to one leg as arms float outward.

Exhale: Circle back to center and alternate sides.

Focus: Flow initiated from the waist (Dantian). 8–10 alternating cycles

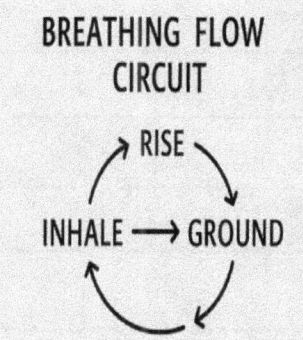

BREATHING FLOW CIRCUIT

RISE

INHALE → GROUND

Each breath lifts energy upward and returns it gently to calm stability.

BODY & WELLBEING BENEFITS

AREA	BODY BENEFIT	DAILY EFFECT
Shoulders & Arms	Improves mobility and blood flow	Eases chronic stiffness
Upper Back & Chest	Expands lung capacity	Freer, deeper breathing
Balance & Coordination	Trains safe body transitions	Smoother daily movement

THERAPEUTIC
Keep elbows soft and wrists light, as if painting air with your hands
Match each motion to your breathing rhythm — not speed.
Small, mindful repetitions are more healing than large ones.

REFLECTION OF THE DAY

- What part of my body began to "flow" today?
- When did I feel the connection between my breath and arms?
- How could this softness change the way I move through daily life?

JOURNAL — My Notes

_____   _____
_____   _____
_____   _____
_____   _____
_____   _____
_____   _____
_____   _____
_____   _____

DAY 5
Gentle knee bend

柔膝屈

Traditional Name: *Rou Xi Qu* — "Soften the Knee Bend"
Focus: To gently strengthen your legs, deepen your connection to the ground, and safely activate circulation without impact.

PREPARATION & BASE BREATHING
Stand (or sit) with feet hip-width apart, shoulders relaxed.
Close your eyes and bring awareness to the soles of your feet.
Inhale: lengthen your spine. Exhale: root your weight evenly through your feet.
Add gentle ankle circles and heel lifts for 4–5 slow rounds.

LEVEL 1 — Bend with Confidence (With Support)
Inhale: Elongate your spine, keeping the crown of the head lifted.
Exhale: Bend your knees gently, as if sitting on the edge of a cloud.
Focus: Light hand contact on chair; move within comfort. 8–10 reps.

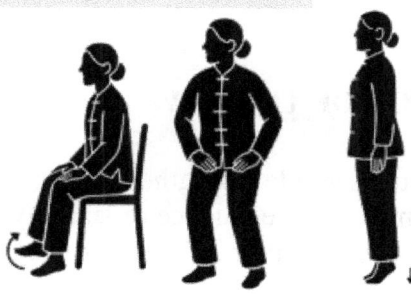
1-Waking Up the Legs

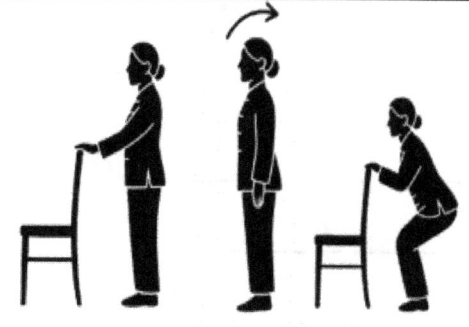
2-Bend with Confidence

LEVEL 2 — Bend with Freedom (Hands Free)
Inhale: Raise arms to chest height, spine upright.
Exhale: Bend knees softly, maintaining balance and calm breath.
Focus: Arms follow the breath; gentle return to center. 10–12 reps.

LEVEL 3 — Bend with Weight Transfer
Inhale: Rise and shift weight slightly to one leg.
Exhale: Bend and center, alternating sides.
Focus: Feel grounding through both feet. 10–12 alternating reps.

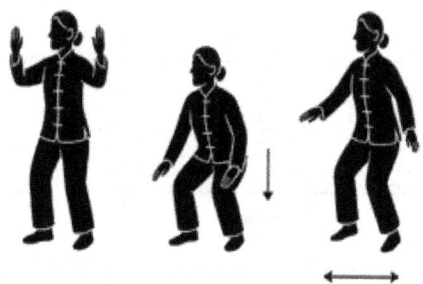
3-Bend with Freedom

BREATHING FLOW CIRCUIT

INHALE → LIFT → EXHALE → GROUND

BODY & WELLBEING BENEFITS

AREA	BODY BENEFIT	DAILY EFFECT
Legs & Hips	Builds functional leg strength	Easier standing, walking, stair climbing
Knees & Joints	Enhances mobility with gentle range	Reduces stiffness, prevents strain
Core & Balance	Improves stability and coordination	Greater confidence in daily movement

THERAPEUTIC TIPS
Keep a chair or wall nearby for safety if needed

Move slowly — precision matters more than depth.

Avoid locking the knees; feel your spine rise with each inhale.

REFLECTION OF THE DAY

- How does gentle strength feel in my legs today?
- Do I notice more balance or stability after bending?
- What does "resilience" mean to me in my everyday steps?

JOURNAL — My Notes

_____   _____

_____   _____

_____   _____

_____   _____

_____   _____

_____   _____

_____   _____

DAY 6
Opening the heart

开心掌

Traditional Name: *Kai Xin Zhang* — "Palms That Open the Heart"
Focus: To release tension in your chest, expand your breathing, and gently invite inner serenity and joy.

PREPARATION & BASE BREATHING
Stand or sit with feet hip-width apart; spine upright; shoulders relaxed.
Place palms at the center of the chest; take **3 slow breaths** into this area.
Rub palms briefly for warmth; rest them on the breastbone for **2 breaths**.
Roll shoulders **backward** ×3, keeping the chest open and neck soft.

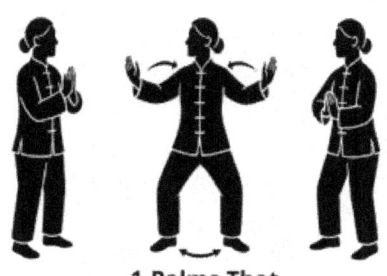

1-Palms That Open the Heart

LEVEL 1 — The Seed Expands (Seated or Standing)
Inhale: Open elbows outward.
Exhale: Return palms to the center.
Focus: Smooth rhythm, relaxed neck. **8–10 cycles.**

LEVEL 2 — Embracing the Horizon
Inhale: Open arms to shoulder height, palms outward.
Exhale: Bring palms together; add soft knee bend.
Focus: Expand from chest center. **8–10 cycles.**

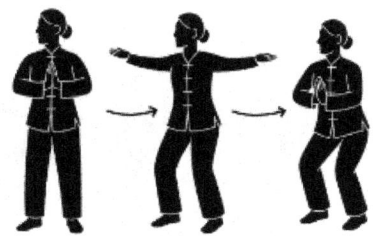

2-Embracing the Horizon

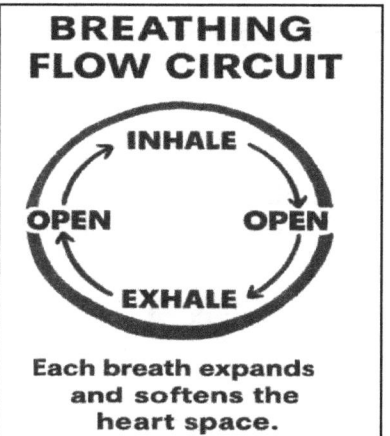

BREATHING FLOW CIRCUIT

INHALE — OPEN — EXHALE — OPEN

Each breath expands and softens the heart space.

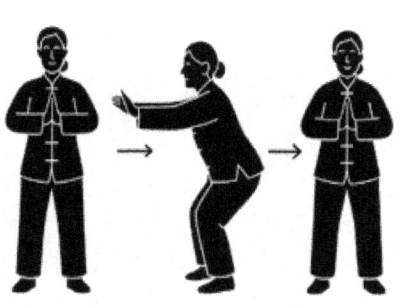

3-Leaning into Trust

LEVEL 3 — Leaning into Trust
Inhale: Open arms; lean slightly forward from hips.
Exhale: Return upright, hands to chest.
Focus: Comfortable range only. **8–10 cycles.**

BODY & WELLBEING BENEFITS

AREA	BODY BENEFIT	DAILY EFFECT
Chest & Upper Back	Gently opens tight chest muscles	Freer, deeper breathing
Shoulders	Softens habitual tension	Lighter posture, easier movement
Emotional Center (Heart Area)	Stimulates calm, soothing pathways	Supports emotional release & inner ease

THERAPEUTIC TIPS
Keep the movement light — think of opening a curtain to let air
Match the arms to your breath, not the other way around.
A small, comfortable range of opening is enough to create change.

REFLECTION OF THE DAY

• What did I feel in my chest when I opened my arms today?

• Was there a softer sigh or a sense of newfound space?

• How would my day change if I brought this "open heart" to my next conversation?

JOURNAL — My Notes

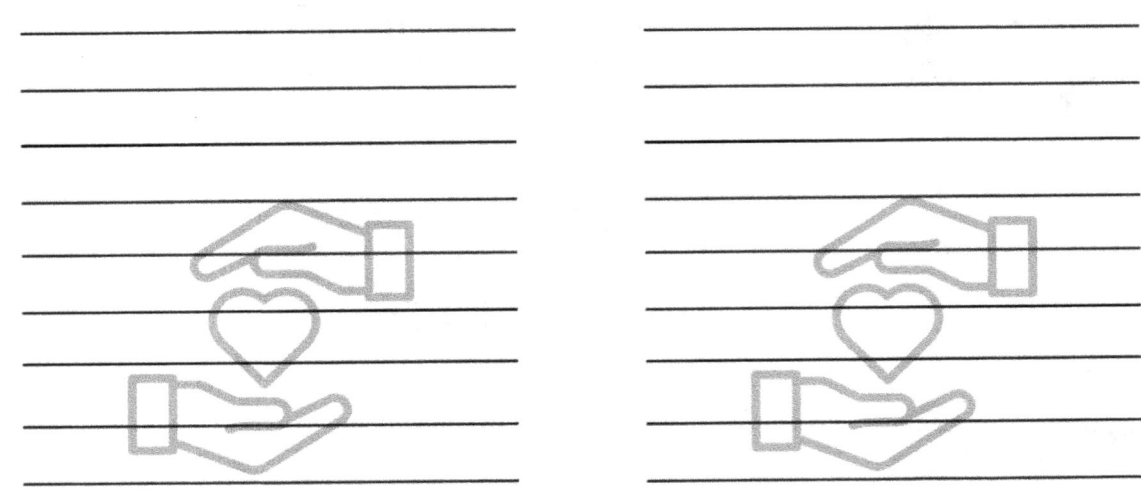

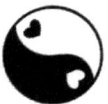

DAY 7
The silence that heals

静坐功
Traditional Name: *Jing Zuo Gong* — "The Practice of Sitting in Stillness"
Focus: To cultivate inner calm, integrate this week's lessons, and reconnect with your inner center of balance and peace.

PREPARATION & BASE BREATHING
Sit with spine upright and feet grounded or legs crossed. Hands rest on thighs or heart–abdomen.
Inhale through nose 4 counts; exhale through mouth 6 counts.
Let breath flow naturally as you observe without controlling it.
Allow the face and shoulders to soften.
Continue 4–6 cycles until the body settles into quiet.

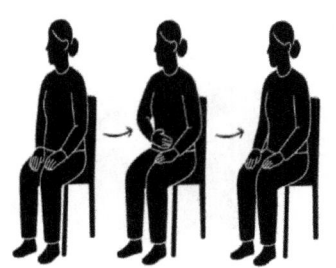

1- Roots in the chair

2- The tree at peace

3- Serene Sway

LEVEL 1 — Roots in the Chair- 8 reps.
Feet flat; notice weight and grounding through the seat.
Observe the natural rise and fall of the abdomen.
Return attention to feet whenever the mind wanders.

LEVEL 2 — The Tree at Peace (Wuji Standing)
Stand with knees soft and arms relaxed by your sides.
Notice small balance adjustments and allow breath to flow freely.
Observe sensations without changing them. 8 reps.

LEVEL 3 — Serene Sway
From Wuji, add a very gentle forward–center rocking.
Inhale to lean slightly toward the toes; exhale to return.
Keep the sway minimal, fluid, and calming. 8 reps.

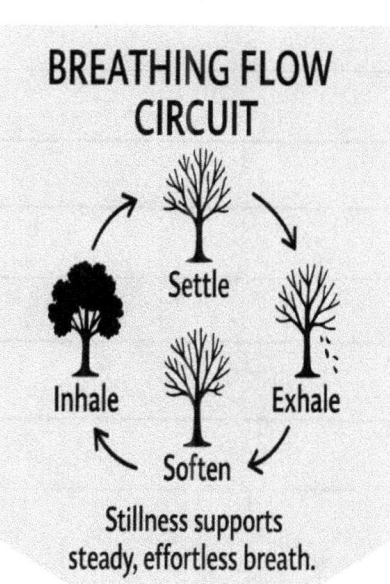

BREATHING FLOW CIRCUIT

Inhale → Settle → Exhale → Soften

Stillness supports steady, effortless breath.

BODY & WELLBEING BENEFITS

AREA	BODY BENEFIT	DAILY EFFECT
Nervous System	Calms overstimulation	More clarity & emotional ease
Posture & Core	Improves alignment awareness	Greater balance & stability
Emotional Center	Encourages inner quiet	Reduced stress reactivity

THERAPEUTIC TIPS
Stillness is active, not rigid — allow micro-movements.
Let breath guide presence, not control.
Thoughts are natural; let them pass like clouds.

REFLECTION OF THE DAY — Week 1 Completion

- What feels slightly different in my body compared to a week ago?
- Which movement made me feel most present?
- How does it feel to begin again, without guilt, when life interrupts practice?

JOURNAL — My Notes

_____   _____
_____   _____
_____   _____
_____   _____
_____   _____
_____   _____
_____   _____

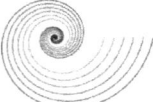

SPECIAL CONCLUSION TO WEEK 1: RECONNECTING

A Major Milestone! You have completed your first week of practice.

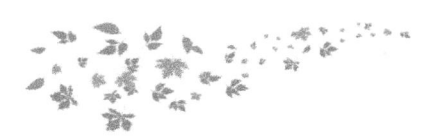

Whether you practiced all 7 days or just a few, what truly matters is that **you took the first step.** That is the most valuable one of all.

This week, you dedicated time to breathe with intention, to move with awareness, and to reconnect with yourself. Maybe you noticed a greater sense of calm, a relief in that persistent tension in your shoulders, or simply the joy of having a moment just for you. Perhaps you only feel the seed of mindfulness, newly planted. **It all counts. Everything is progress.**

I invite you to reflect (you can write it in your journal):

- What new or different sensation does your body feel today, compared to a week ago?
- Of all the movements you learned, which one made you feel most present or that you enjoyed the most?
- What emotion visited you most often during your practice? Was it tranquility, curiosity, a little frustration, or perhaps gratitude?

If you have the "Practice Journal," this is the perfect time to write down your impressions.

And if life kept you from completing some days, remember this with kindness: **Tai Chi is not a race; it's a circular journey, like the seasons.** It's not about "catching up," but about "beginning again." Every time you return to your practice, you do so from a new place, with a deeper understanding.

Rest, integrate, and celebrate yourself. I'll see you tomorrow, with renewed energy, to begin Week 2: STRENGTHENING.

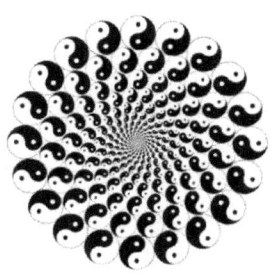

I invite you to reflect on your first week

This is your time with yourself

CHAPTER 4 -WEEK 2-Strengthen
Day 8-The pilar of strength

定体力

Traditional Name: *Ding Ti Li* — "Stability of the Body's Power"
Focus: To activate legs, center, and balance so you can feel grounded, strong, and confident in your everyday movements.

> **PREPARATION & BASE BREATHING**
> Sit or stand with a long spine; feet grounded and knees soft.
> Let shoulders drop and bring awareness to legs, feet, or sitting points.
> Sway gently side to side, then let movement fade.
> Circle shoulders back ×3 and forward ×3.
> Place hands on lower belly; inhale to widen, exhale to draw inward ×3.

LEVEL 1 —Building the pillar
Press feet gently into the ground as you inhale, awakening legs and lower belly.
Exhale to engage the center with a light inward draw.
Optional: add small heel lifts on the inhale and lower on the exhale. Repeat 8 cycles.

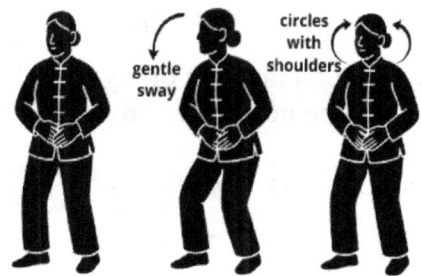
1-Building the Pillar

LEVEL 2 — The Grounded Rise
Inhale to lift arms to chest height (standing or seated).
Exhale into a light squat or small forward lean from the hips. Inhale to return upright, lowering arms with control. Repeat 8 cycles.

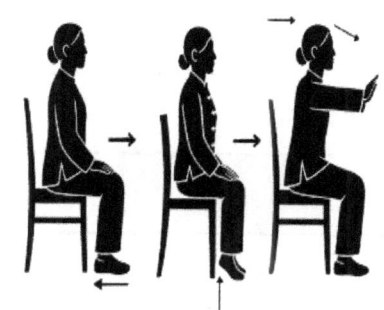
2-The Grounded Rise

LEVEL 3 — Power Flow (Light Resistance)
Hold a light object at the chest; inhale to extend arms forward.
Exhale to bring it back while gently straightening legs or engaging the center.
Optional: add heel lifts or grounded foot presses for deeper activation. Repeat 8 cycles.

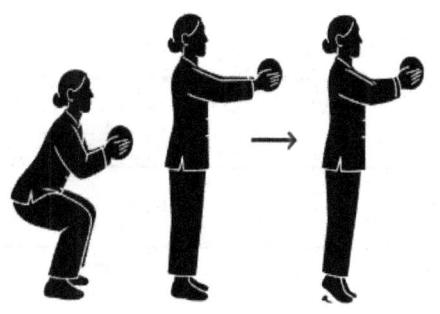
3-Power Flow (With Light Resistance)

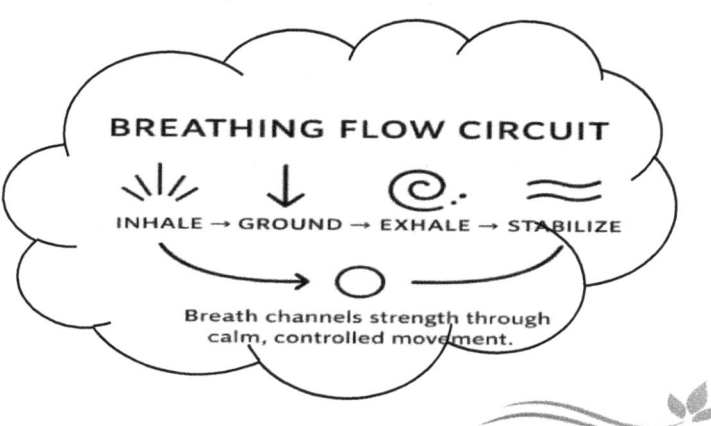

BREATHING FLOW CIRCUIT
INHALE → GROUND → EXHALE → STABILIZE
Breath channels strength through calm, controlled movement.

BODY & WELLBEING BENEFITS

AREA	BODY BENEFIT	DAILY EFFECT
Legs & Hips	Strengthens foundational muscles	More stable walking & standing
Core	Activates deep abdominal support	Greater confidence in movement
Joints	Trains controlled bending	Safer transitions in daily tasks

THERAPEUTIC TIPS
Keep movements small and pain-free.
Prioritize grounding over intensity.
Let breath lead the effort, not force.

REFLECTION OF THE DAY
- When did I feel my legs or my core "awaken"?
- What does "being strong and stable" mean to me at this stage of my life?

JOURNAL — My Notes

_____   _____
_____   _____
_____   _____
_____   _____
_____   _____
_____   _____
_____   _____

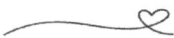

DAY 9
The power beneath the surface

内劲行

Traditional Name: *Nei Jin Xing* — "Walking with Inner Force"
Focus: To activate the deeper muscles of your hips, legs, and core while refining your balance, so each step feels more controlled and supported from within.

PREPARATION & BASE BREATHING
Sit or stand tall with feet grounded and knees soft.
Breathe in 4 counts, out 6 counts ×3, letting shoulders soften.
Shift weight gently side to side, then pause in stillness.
Hands on lower belly; take 3 slow breaths to awaken your center.

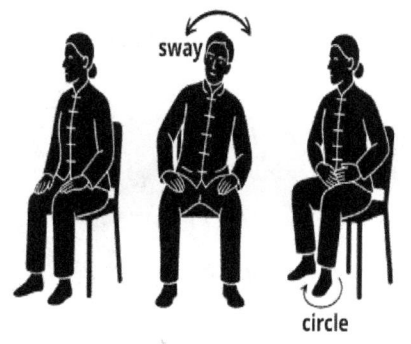

1-Stepping from Your Center

LEVEL 1 — Stepping from your center. Repeat 8 cycles.
Inhale to lengthen posture; exhale to lift one foot or knee slightly.
Lower on the inhale and change sides with steady rhythm.
Optional: swing the opposite arm gently as if walking.

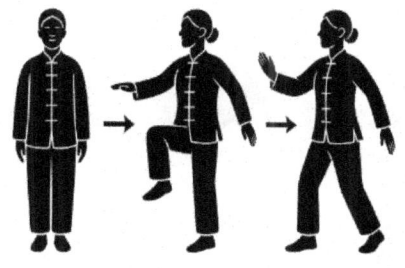

2-Safe step

LEVEL 2 — Forward Shift
Step one foot forward (or slide it forward if seated).
Inhale to shift weight toward the front; exhale to return.
Switch legs, keeping torso upright and relaxed. Repeat 8 cycles.

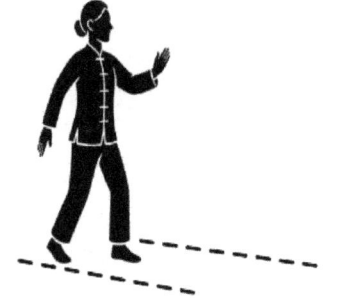

3-Inner Strength Walk

LEVEL 3 — Inner Strength Walk. Repeat 8 cycles.
Walk slowly in a straight line, starting each step from the hip.
Inhale as the leg floats forward; exhale as the foot grounds with control.
Move as if through water—fluid, balanced, intentional.

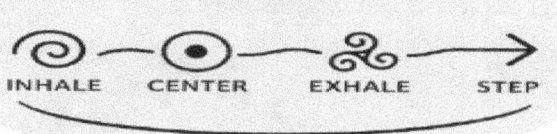

BREATHING FLOW CIRCUIT
INHALE — CENTER — EXHALE — STEP

BODY & WELLBEING BENEFITS

AREA	BODY BENEFIT	DAILY EFFECT
Hips & Legs	Strengthens walking muscles	Safer, smoother steps
Knees & Ankles	Trains controlled shifting	Better balance & stability
Core	Improves postural support	More confidence in movement

THERAPEUTIC TIPS
Keep steps small and slow.
Allow breath to guide weight shifts.
Use a wall or chair for safety if needed.

REFLECTION OF THE DAY

• How did it feel to "move from within" today?
• In what moment this week would I like to remember this centered way of walking?

JOURNAL — My Notes

DAY 10

The core that carries you

丹田功

Traditional Name: *Dan Tian Gong* — "Cultivating the Power Center"
Focus: To strengthen the deep abdominal and pelvic muscles by connecting to your energetic center—the Dantian—so every movement feels more stable and supported.

PREPARATION & BASE BREATHING
Sit or stand tall with feet grounded and knees soft.
Hands on lower belly; inhale to expand gently into your palms.
Exhale to soften the belly and settle your weight downward.

Raise arms with an inhale, lower with an exhale ×3, then return hands to center.

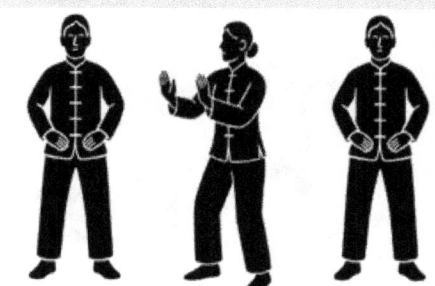

1-Awakening Your Inner Engine

LEVEL 1 — Your inner engine. Repeat 8 cycles.
Inhale to lengthen spine; exhale to draw belly inward with light activation.
Add a small hinge forward (standing) or grounded foot press (seated).
Return upright on the inhale, keeping movements soft and controlled.

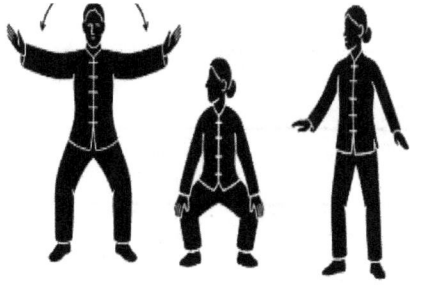

2-Centered Squat

LEVEL 2 — Centered Squat. Repeat 8 cycles.
Inhale to lift arms to shoulder height.
Exhale into a shallow squat or forward lean, engaging the low belly.
Inhale to rise back up with steady feet and relaxed shoulders.

LEVEL 3 — Spiral Core Activation. Repeat 8 cycles.
Inhale to lift arms in front of the chest.
Exhale to rotate the torso gently to one side, hips steady.
Inhale to center, then rotate to the other side with ease.

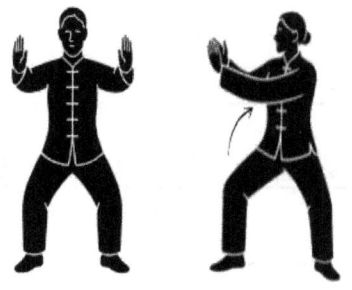

3-Spiral Core Activation

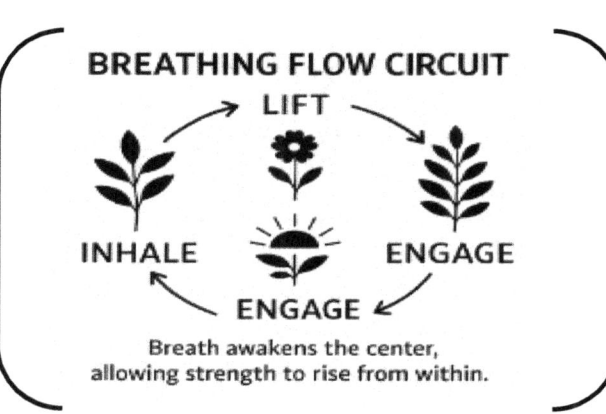

BREATHING FLOW CIRCUIT
LIFT — INHALE — ENGAGE — ENGAGE
Breath awakens the center, allowing strength to rise from within.

BODY & WELLBEING BENEFITS

AREA	BODY BENEFIT	DAILY EFFECT
Core & Abdomen	Activates deep stabilizing muscles	Safer bending & standing
Hips & Lower Back	Supports spine alignment	Less strain during daily tasks
Posture	Encourages upright, balanced stance	Greater energy & confidence

THERAPEUTIC TIPS

Engage the center gently—never brace or hold breath.
Keep movements small and fluid.
Imagine warmth gathering in the lower belly (Dantian).

REFLECTION OF THE DAY

- How did it feel to move from my center instead of from tension?
- What does "living from my center" mean to me today?

JOURNAL — My Notes

_____   _____
_____   _____
_____   _____
_____   _____
_____   _____
_____   _____
_____   _____

◆◆◆

DAY 11
The hips that hold you

胯开功

Traditional Name: *Kua Kai Gong* — "Opening the Hip Gate"
Focus: To unlock and strengthen your hips by activating your glutes, stabilizer muscles, and the connection between your legs and core. Today you train the foundation of your balance, power, and fluidity.

PREPARATION & BASE BREATHING
Sit or stand tall with feet grounded and knees soft.
Hands on hips; inhale through the nose, exhale softly through the mouth.
With each exhale, feel the hips settle, soften, and gently open from within.
Make small hip circles and slow side-to-side sways to awaken the area.

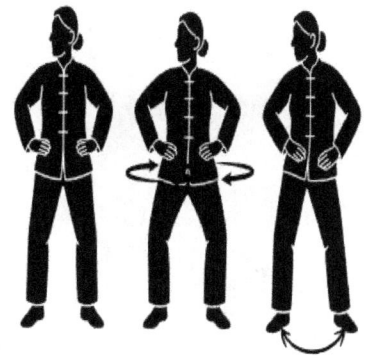
1-Opening the Hip Gate

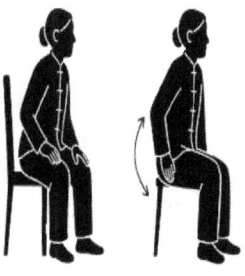
2-Seated Hip Walk

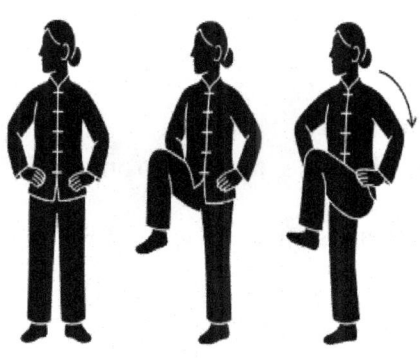
3-Open Gate Step

LEVEL 1 — Opening the hip gate
Inhale to lengthen spine; exhale to slide one hip slightly forward.
Return to center and switch sides with slow, steady "steps."
Let glutes and low belly engage without strain. Do 8 cycles.

LEVEL 2 — Seated hip walk. Do 8 cycles
Stand or sit tall; inhale at center.
Exhale to pulse one hip outward, return to center, then switch sides.
Keep abdomen lightly engaged and movements small and controlled.

LEVEL 3 — Open Gate Step. Do 8 cycles.
Lift one knee; exhale to gently open it outward like a swinging gate.
Return to center with control and alternate legs.
Keep torso steady as the hip joint moves and activates.

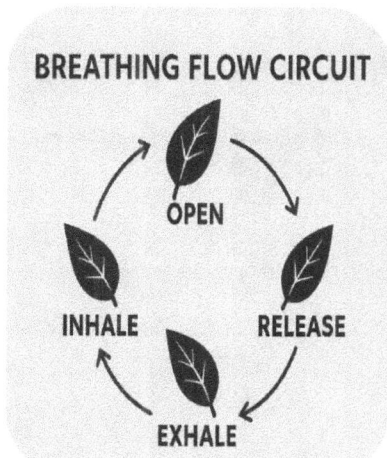
BREATHING FLOW CIRCUIT

BODY & WELLBEING BENEFITS

AREA	BODY BENEFIT	DAILY EFFECT
Hips	Improves mobility and joint lubrication	Safer, smoother steps
Lower Back	Reduces tension & compensations	Less stiffness during daily tasks
Balance	Enhances weight-shift control	Greater stability when walking

THERAPEUTIC TIPS

If one side feels tighter, move smaller—not deeper.
Keep the core gently engaged for hip support.
Aim for smooth, circular motion instead of force.

REFLECTION OF THE DAY

- How did it feel to move from my hips today?

- What "door" in my life am I ready to gently open?

JOURNAL — My Notes

DAY 12
The power of your step

步法功
Traditional Name: *Bu Fa Gong* — "Skillful Stepping Method"
Focus: To build strength and confidence through intentional stepping, improving weight transfer, leg and glute activation, and your ability to move forward with stability and purpo

PREPARATION & BASE BREATHING
Sit or stand tall with feet grounded and knees soft.
Breathe in 4 counts, out 6 counts ×3, feeling steady beneath your feet.
Shift weight gently side-to-side, awakening hips and ankles.
Make small ankle circles, then finish with light heel lifts.

LEVEL 1 — Step Activation
Inhale to prepare; exhale to slide one foot forward (seated) or take a small step (standing).
Inhale to return and switch legs with steady rhythm.
Optional: add opposite arm swing to simulate walking. Repeat 8 cycles.

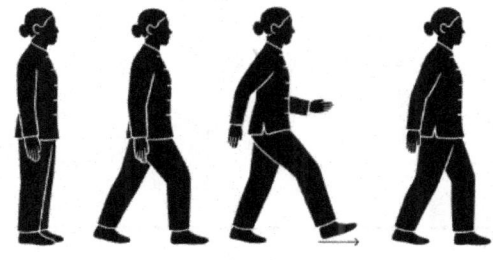
1-Step Activation

LEVEL 2 — Intentional Step
Step one foot forward; inhale to grow tall over both legs.
Exhale to settle weight into the front foot, then inhale to return.
Switch legs, keeping posture upright and core gently engaged. Repeat 8 cycles.

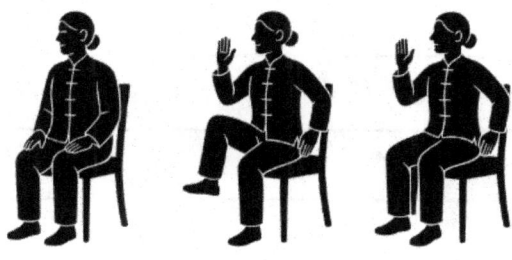
2-Intentional Step

LEVEL 3 — Rooted Walk
Walk slowly in a straight line, beginning each step from the hip.
Inhale as the leg initiates; exhale as the foot lands with control.
Maintain a calm, steady rhythm (seated: walk in place with arm–leg coordination). Repeat 8 cycles.

3-Rooted Walk

BREATHING FLOW CIRCUIT

INHALE → PREPARE → EXHALE STEP

↻ *Breath slows the pace, helping each step land with balance and intention.*

BODY & WELLBEING BENEFITS

AREA	BODY BENEFIT	DAILY EFFECT
Hips & Legs	Strengthens stepping muscles	Safer, more confident walking
Ankles	Improves mobility & stability	Reduces risk of stumbles
Whole Body	Trains mindful weight-shifting	Steady transitions & turning

THERAPEUTIC TIPS
Keep steps small and controlled.
Let breath set the rhythm.
Use support if needed—safety first.

REFLECTION OF THE DAY

- How did it feel to walk more slowly and intentionally today?
- Was there a moment when your breath and movement became one?
- What "next step" do I want to take in my life?

JOURNAL — My Notes

_____   _____

_____   _____

_____   _____

_____   _____

_____   _____

_____   _____

_____   _____

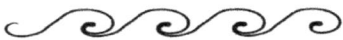

DAY 13
The strength that bends

柔力功

Traditional Name: *Rou Li Gong* — "The Power of Softness"
Focus: To build strength and flexibility through flowing, spiral movements that awaken your core, hips, and spine. This is not rigid strength—it is rooted, responsive strength that can bend without breaking.

PREPARATION & BASE BREATHING
Sit or stand tall with feet grounded and knees soft.
Inhale through the nose, exhale through the mouth ×3.
Imagine bamboo: rooted, flexible, bending without breaking.
Lift arms in soft arcs, then make small torso circles to awaken the spine.

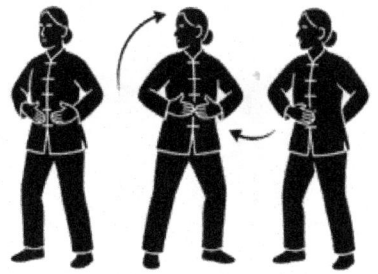
1-Flow Circles

LEVEL 1 — Flow Circles Do 8 cycles.
Inhale to gently spiral the torso to one side.
Exhale to return to center, then switch sides.
Let the waist and spine lead while hips stay steady.

LEVEL 2 — Spiral Squat Do 8 cycles.
Exhale into a shallow squat while rotating to one side.
Inhale to rise back to center and alternate sides.
Keep the core lightly active and arms flowing with the turn.

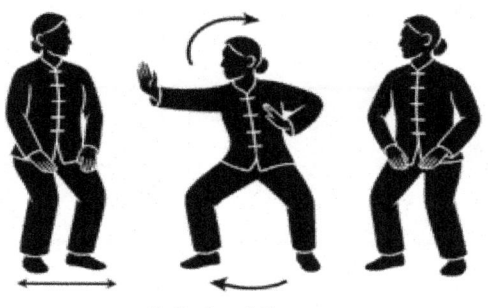
2-Spiral Squat

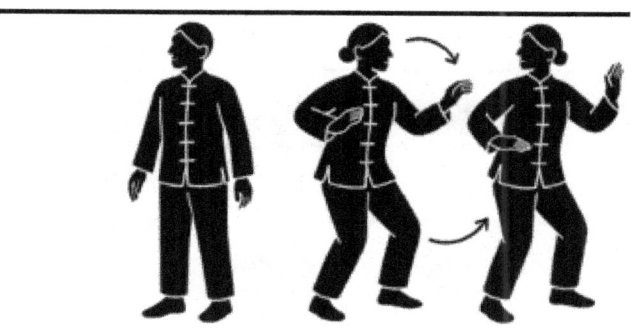
3-Wave Step

LEVEL 3 — Wave Step
Step to the side as your torso follows in a soft wave.
Arms move in an easy arc; return to center and switch sides.
Maintain one continuous, gentle motion.
Repeat 8 cycles.

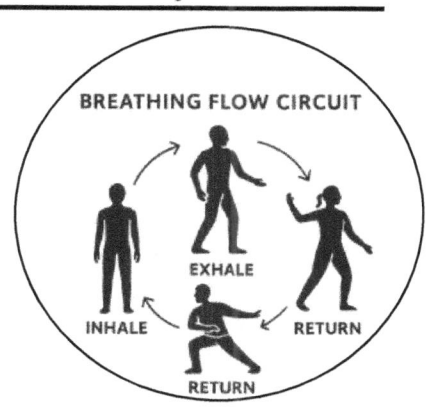

BODY & WELLBEING BENEFITS

AREA	BODY BENEFIT	DAILY EFFECT
Spine & Waist	Improves rotation & flexibility	Easier bending & reaching
Hips	Encourages smooth lateral movement	Safer side-stepping
Back & Shoulders	Reduces stiffness & tension	Freer daily turning

THERAPEUTIC TIPS
Move as if water were guiding you.
Keep hips relaxed but grounded.
Small spirals are more effective—and safer
— than large ones.

REFLECTION OF THE DAY

- What did it feel like to move in spirals and waves today?

- Did any part of me feel freer afterward?

JOURNAL — My Notes

_____   _____

_____   _____

_____   _____

_____   _____

_____   _____

_____   _____

_____   _____

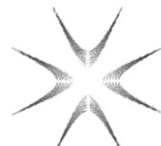

DAY 14
The to stay, the readiness to shift

站桩易动
Traditional Name: *Zhan Zhuang Yi Dong* — "Stillness Becoming Movement"
Focus: To integrate the strength of your core, hips, and legs in a posture that is still on the outside but quietly ready to move on the inside.

PREPARATION & BASE BREATHING
Sit or stand tall with feet grounded and knees soft.
Inhale through the nose, exhale through the mouth ×3.
Shift gently side to side, sensing your base becoming steady.
Place hands on lower belly; breathe into a calm, strong center.

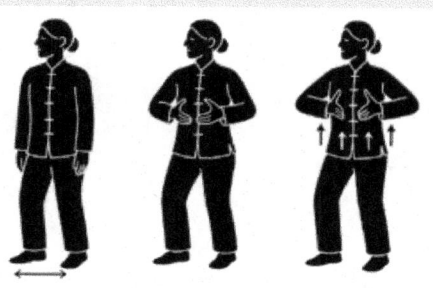
1-Power Hold

LEVEL 1 — Power Hold
Lift arms as if cradling a soft ball; engage legs and belly gently.
Hold the position with alert stillness, then rest briefly.
Repeat for 8 cycles.

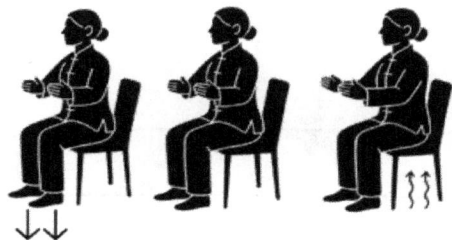
2-Root and Release

LEVEL 2 — Root and Release
Bend into a shallow squat or press feet firmly if seated.
Hold 10–15 seconds with upright posture and engaged center.
Exhale to release smoothly before repeating.

LEVEL 3 — Fluid Transition
Step slowly forward or sideways with breath-led control.
Return to center on an inhale, maintaining steady alignment.
Alternate sides, practicing movement without losing your base. Repeat 8 cycles.

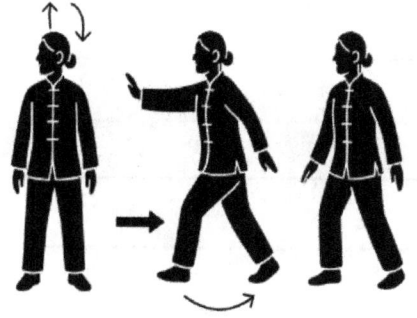
3-Fluid Transition

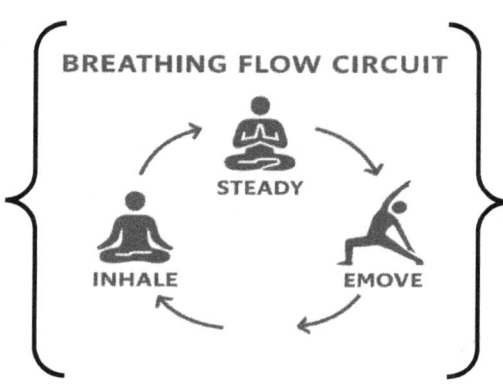

BODY & WELLBEING BENEFITS

AREA	BODY BENEFIT	DAILY EFFECT
Thighs & Hips	Builds foundational strength	Easier standing & direction changes
Core	Supports upright posture	Greater stability in stillness
Balance	Trains safe transitions	Reduces hesitation when moving

THERAPEUTIC TIPS
Strength can be soft—never force the holds.
Keep knees comfortably bent, not locked.
Move only when the breath invites the transition.

REFLECTION OF THE DAY

- Where do I need to stay strong without becoming tense?

- How did it feel to be still on the outside but ready on the inside?

JOURNAL — My Notes

_____   _____
_____   _____
_____   _____
_____   _____
_____   _____
_____   _____
_____   _____

SPECIAL CONCLUSION TO WEEK 2: STRENGTHENING

A Foundation Built from Within.

Congratulations on completing Week 2 of your journey — seven days of planting deeper roots, activating your body, and reinforcing your inner pillar of stability.

Perhaps you've noticed your legs feeling more grounded, your hips more aware, your center more present. Maybe you stood a little taller, held your breath a little calmer, carried yourself with a hint of new confidence. Even simply showing up — in spite of fatigue, distraction or doubt — is a real victory.

This week wasn't just about movement. It was about embodied strength.
You've started to build the infrastructure of your well-being, a base that will support everything you do—today and tomorrow.

Reflect in your "Inner Journey Notebook":
- Which movement of the week made you feel most empowered, most connected to your body?
- In what way has your relationship with your legs, your hips, or your core changed?
- What sense of strength did you begin to cultivate—physical, emotional, or perhaps both?

If you missed a day, or two — be kind to yourself. Strength is not built through perfection; it is built through returning, through consistency, through presence. Every time you come back to your practice, you add one more layer to your foundation, one more thread to your strength.

Now, take these next few days to integrate what you've built. Let your body rest, absorb, and organize itself. Prepare your mind for what's coming: **Week 3 – BALANCING**, where you'll flow between strength and ease, poise and motion, groundedness and shift.

Sit with this: You are stronger than yesterday. Your base is deeper. The path ahead is open.

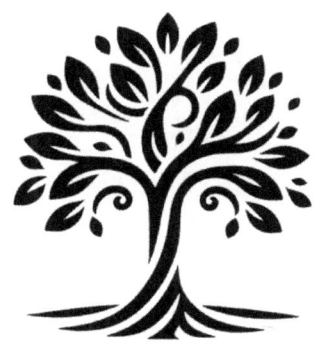

I invite you to reflect on your first week

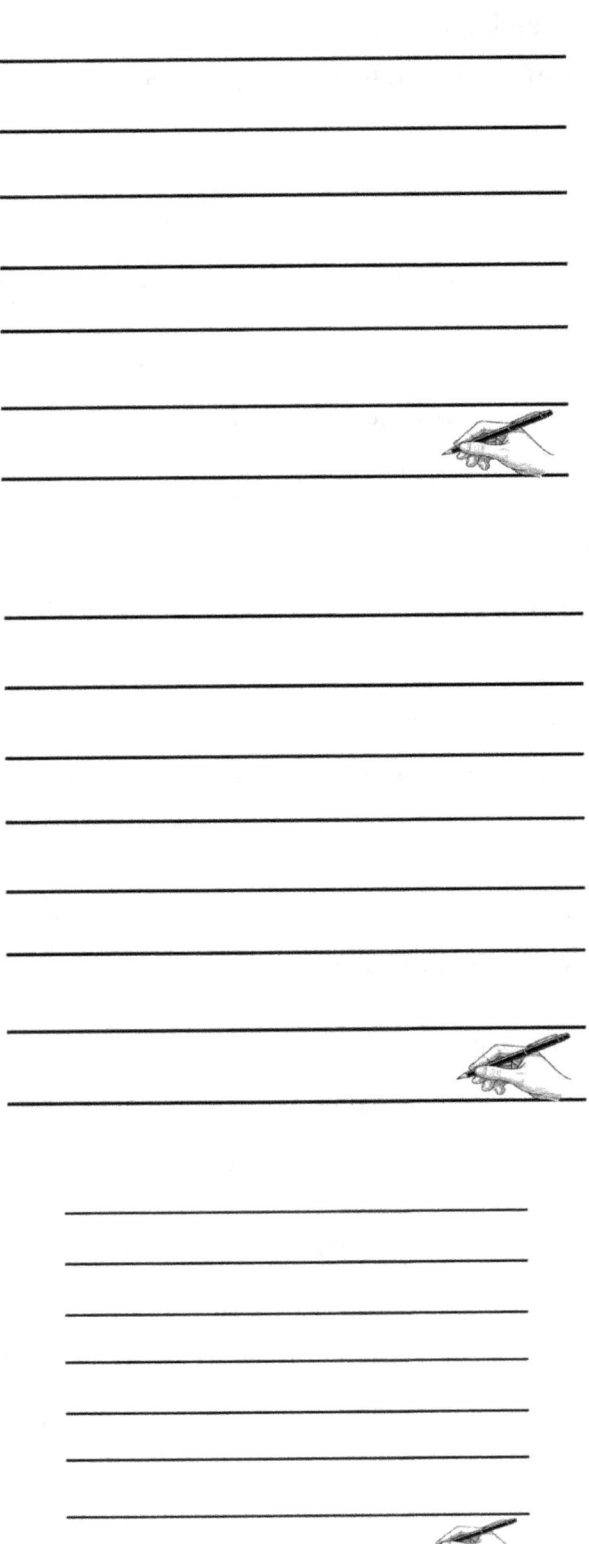

This is your time with yourself

CHAPTER 5 -WEEK 3-Expand
Day 15-The of stillness and motion

环静功

Traditional Name: *Huan Jing Gong* — "Circling Stillness"
Focus: To cultivate dynamic balance by alternating between stillness and subtle motion, activating your center, legs, and hips while your body stabilizes and transitions with ease.

PREPARATION & BASE BREATHING
Sit or stand tall with feet grounded and knees soft.
Shift gently side-to-side, awakening your base.
Circle ankles and wrists slowly in both directions.
Hands on lower belly; inhale to widen, exhale to draw in.

LEVEL 1 — Circles stillness
Inhale to shift weight gently to one side (standing or seated).
Exhale to return to center, then switch sides smoothly.
Repeat soft sways, allowing subtle and steady transitions. For 8 cycles.

LEVEL 2 — Steady-Step Balance. Repeat 8 cycles.
Step or slide one foot to the side with slow control.
Shift weight onto that foot, keeping spine tall and core engaged.
Return to center and alternate sides with calm rhythm.

LEVEL 3 — Flowing Transition Repeat 8 cycles.
Trace a curved path with forward, diagonal, and side steps.
Inhale to begin each direction; exhale to settle into the step.
Move like a gentle arc, returning to center with ease.

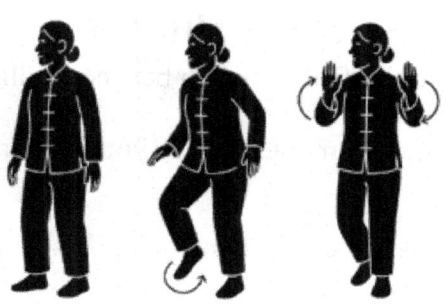

1-Circling Stillness

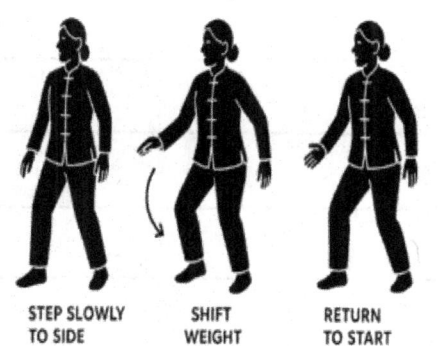

STEP SLOWLY TO SIDE — SHIFT WEIGHT — RETURN TO START

2-Steady-Step Balance

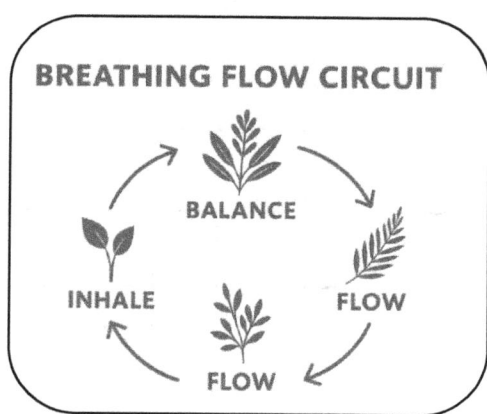

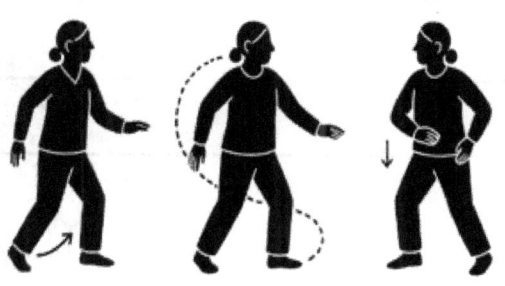

3-Flowing Transition

BODY & WELLBEING BENEFITS

AREA	BODY BENEFIT	DAILY EFFECT
Hips & Legs	Improves weight-shift control	Safer turning & stepping sideways
Core	Enhances midline stability	Better balance in daily transitions
Ankles	Builds mobility & support	Reduced wobbling and hesitation

THERAPEUTIC TIPS
Keep transitions soft—no sharp or rushed movements.
Let breath determine the pace.
Small curves are safer and more effective than large steps.

REFLECTION OF THE DAY

- How did it feel to switch between stillness and movement?

- Was there a moment when you felt particularly stable… or challenged?

JOURNAL — My Notes

DAY 16
The center that moves with you

中定功

Traditional Name: *Zhong Ding Gong* — "Cultivating Central Equilibrium"
Focus: To develop a stable, responsive center so you can stay grounded while you move, turn, or change dire

PREPARATION & BASE BREATHING
Sit or stand tall with feet grounded and knees soft.
Shift weight side-to-side to awaken your base.
Rotate torso gently, keeping hips steady and breath smooth.
Hands on lower belly; inhale to expand, exhale to settle inward.

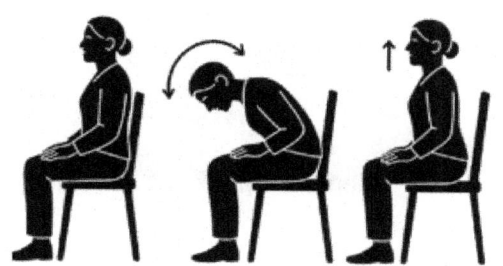
1-Moving Around Your Axis

LEVEL 1 —Moving around your axis
Inhale to lengthen spine; exhale to lean slightly forward (seated) or toward the balls of the feet (standing).
Inhale to return to center with even weight.
Repeat gentle front–back shifts with a calm, steady axis. For 8 cycles.

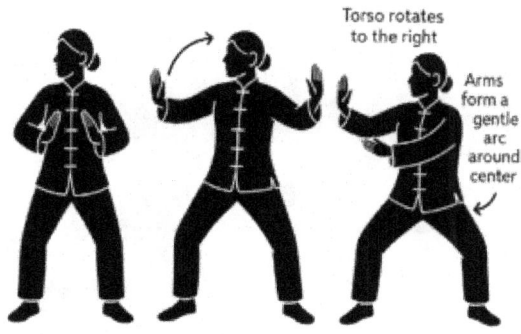
2-Rotating Arms

LEVEL 2 — Rotating Arms Around Center
Inhale to raise arms to chest height.
Exhale to rotate torso right or left, hips steady and core engaged.
Return to center on the inhale, moving smoothly from the spine. For 8 cycles.

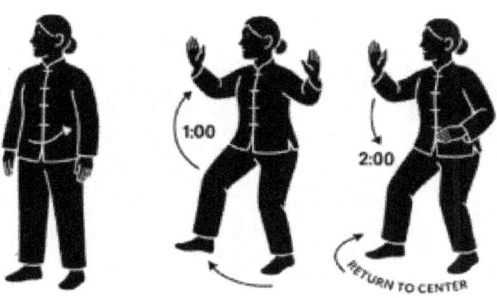
3-Compass Step

LEVEL 3 — Compass Step Around Center
Take a small diagonal or side step, initiating from the center.
Exhale to place the foot and settle weight without collapsing.
Return to neutral, repeating gentle compass steps around your axis. Repeat 8 cycles.

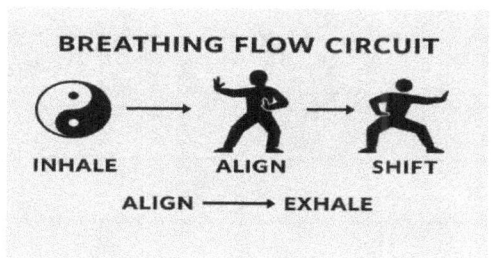
BREATHING FLOW CIRCUIT
INHALE → ALIGN → SHIFT
ALIGN ⟶ EXHALE

BODY & WELLBEING BENEFITS

AREA	BODY BENEFIT	DAILY EFFECT
Core & Waist	Strengthens central control	Safer turning & bending
Hips	Trains steady shifting	More stable weight transfer
Whole Body	Supports directional changes	Reduces wobbling & overcompensation

THERAPEUTIC TIPS

Imagine a line from crown to lower belly guiding all movement.
Keep steps small and hips softened.
Let breath determine when to shift and when to return.

REFLECTION OF THE DAY

- How did it feel to move around my center today?

- When did it feel most grounded… or most challenging?

- Where in my life do I want to recall this feeling of a stable center when "turning" or "changing direction"?

JOURNAL — My Notes

DAY 17
The bridge between points

桥接功

Traditional Name: *Qiao Jie Gong* — "Bridging the Connective Path"

Focus: To explore how your body creates a bridge—between ground and space, stillness and motion—by connecting legs, core, and upper body in a coordinated flow.

PREPARATION & BASE BREATHING
Sit or stand tall, grounding your feet or sitting bones.
Press lightly through toes and heels to awaken your base.
Roll shoulders back and forward, softening ribs on each exhale.
Hands on upper belly: inhale to expand, exhale to release tension.

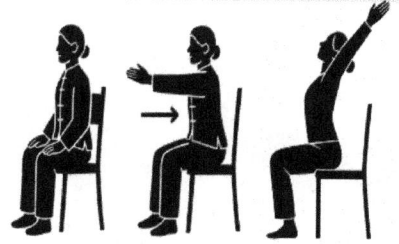

1-Simple Bridge Shift

LEVEL 1 — Simple Bridge Shift. 8 cycles.
Shift gently forward, letting arms float ahead as feet (or sitting bones) support you.
Shift slightly back, allowing arms to move behind without collapsing.
Repeat soft forward–back shifts, staying steady through the center.

LEVEL 2 — Diagonal Reach Bridge
Step or slide one foot diagonally while the opposite arm reaches across and upward.
Return to center on the inhale, switching sides smoothly and with control.
Feel a diagonal "bridge" connecting foot, core, and reaching hand. For 8 cycles.

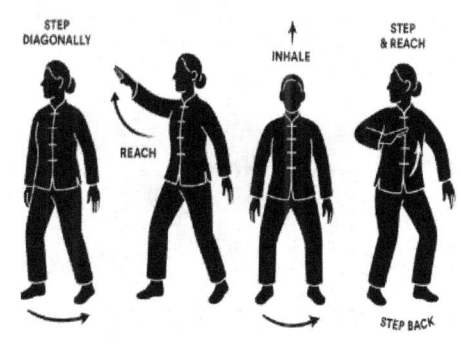

2-Diagonal Reach Bridge

LEVEL 3 — Flowing Bridge Walk

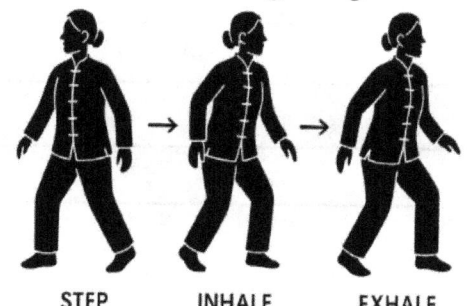

3-Flowing Bridge Walk

Walk (or trace with your feet) a gentle diagonal pattern: forward-right, sideways-left, center.
Inhale to begin each step; exhale to settle weight before changing direction.
Let torso and arms follow the path so the whole body connects as one. Repeat 8 cycles.

BREATHING FLOW CIRCUIT

INHALE → CONNECT → EXHALE → FLOW

BODY & WELLBEING BENEFITS

AREA	BODY BENEFIT	DAILY EFFECT
Feet–Core Line	Improves coordination and connection	Smoother walking & turning
Hips & Torso	Enhances diagonal stability	Easier reaching across body (cinturón, estantes)
Whole Body	Integrates movement into one system	Less imbalance, fewer "disjointed" motions

THERAPEUTIC TIPS
Imagine your body as a bridge—stable, flexible, and connected.
Keep your steps small to maintain smooth coordination.
Let the exhale guide the moment you settle into each step.

REFLECTION OF THE DAY

- Where did I feel the "bridge" most clearly—my feet, hips, torso, or arms?
- Was there a moment when my whole body moved as one unified whole?
- In what area of my life do I want to build a "bridge" between who I was and what is coming?

JOURNAL — My Notes

DAY 18
The weight that's light

轻重功

Traditional Name: Qian Zhong Gong– "Mastering Lightness and Heaviness"
Focus: Explore the contrast of weight and lightness so you can carry, shift, and release your body's mass with ease. Strength in the legs and core, clarity in movement, and freedom in posture.

PREPARATION & BASE BREATHING
Sit or stand tall with feet grounded and knees soft.
Shift weight gently side-to-side to awaken your base.
Lift heels or toes lightly, sensing where your weight settles.
Hands on lower belly; inhale to rise, exhale to sink and ground.

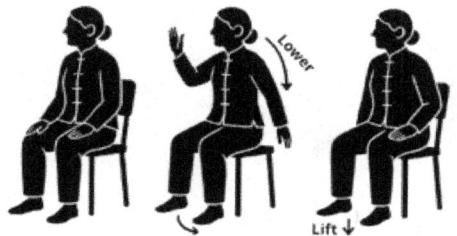
1-Strong Base

LEVEL 1 — Light Heels, Strong Base- 8 cycles
Inhale to prepare; exhale to lift heels slightly (seated or standing).
Hold a brief sense of lightness before lowering with control.
Repeat small lifts, keeping your center quietly engaged.

LEVEL 2 — Guided Weight Shift- 8 cycles
Step or slide one foot forward and inhale at center.
Exhale to shift weight onto the front foot, noticing heaviness move.
Inhale to return to neutral, alternating sides with smooth control.

LEVEL 3 — Floating Steps- 8 cycles
Walk slowly in a straight line or mimic steps while seated.
Inhale as the foot lifts into lightness; exhale as it settles onto the ground.
Pause softly before each landing, sensing the transition of weight.

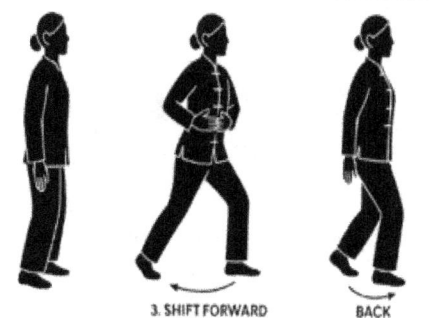
2-Guided Weight Shift

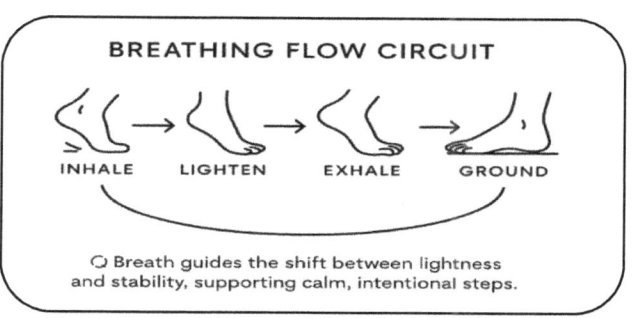
3-Floating Steps

BODY & WELLBEING BENEFITS

AREA	BODY BENEFIT	DAILY EFFECT
Feet & Ankles	Strengthens stabilizing muscles	Safer walking & standing
Hips & Legs	Improves weight transfer	More control in small spaces
Whole Body	Coordinates breath with footwork	Reduced fatigue & wobbling

THERAPEUTIC TIPS
Let the heel rise be small — subtle work builds deeper stability.
Feel the difference between light (lifting) and heavy (settling).
Keep shoulders soft so the legs can do the balancing work.

REFLECTION OF THE DAY

- When did I feel "lightness" most clearly?
- When did grounding feel supportive instead of heavy?
- Where in my life do I need more grounding — and where more lightness?

JOURNAL — My Notes

_____   _____
_____   _____
_____   _____
_____   _____
_____   _____
_____   _____
_____   _____

DAY 19
The balance beneath you

根地功

Traditional Name: Gen Di Gong — "Rooting to the Ground"
Focus: To deepen your balance by strengthening your connection to the ground. You work through feet, ankles and hips (or your seated base) so stability comes not from freezing, but from rooting with awareness.

PREPARATION & BASE BREATHING
Stand or sit tall with feet (or hips) grounded and knees soft.
Close your eyes; inhale to feel the body rise lightly.
Exhale to let your weight sink calmly into the floor or chair.
Repeat 3 slow breaths, sensing a steady, supportive base beneath you.

LEVEL 1 — Foot & Ankle Circles
Circle one ankle slowly while keeping your upper body relaxed.
Shift a little weight and repeat on the other foot, lifting the heel softly.
Place both hands on your lower belly and breathe, sensing warmth and steadiness. For 8 cycles.

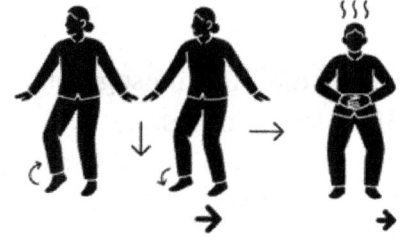

1-Foot and ankle circles

LEVEL 2 — Stepping Root
Step slightly forward or to the side; inhale at center.
Exhale to press into the stepping foot, feeling the ground respond.
Return to neutral and repeat, keeping steps small and steady. Repeat 8 cycles.

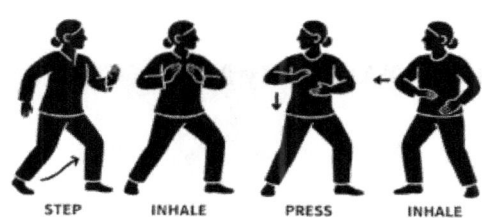

2-Stepping Root

LEVEL 3 — Root Flow
Take a small diagonal step; inhale to move the foot, exhale to root your weight.
Return to center with calm control, switching sides each round.
Repeat slow diagonal steps, sensing grounding through every placement. For 8 cycles.

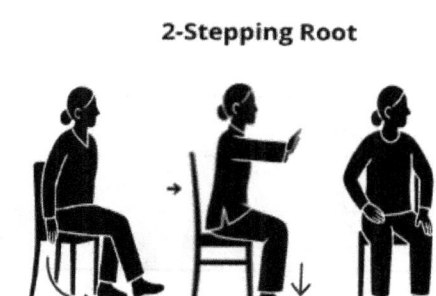

3-Root Flow

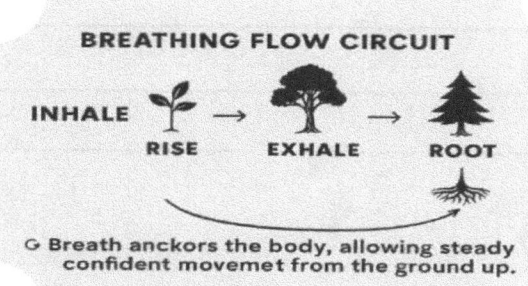

BREATHING FLOW CIRCUIT
INHALE — RISE → EXHALE — TREE → ROOT
Breath anckors the body, allowing steady confident movemet from the ground up.

BODY & WELLBEING BENEFITS

AREA	BODY BENEFIT	DAILY EFFECT
Feet & Ankles	Strengthens stabilizers	Safer walking & turning
Knees & Hips	Improves joint support	More confident weight shifts
Whole Body	Enhances grounded balance	Reduces fear of falling

THERAPEUTIC TIPS
Think of your feet as roots gently gripping the earth.
Keep steps small so grounding remains calm and controlled.
Let the exhale guide each moment of settling into your base.

REFLECTION OF THE DAY

- When today did I feel most grounded—during stillness or movement?
- How did rooting through my feet or base affect my confidence?
- In which part of my life would stronger "roots" bring more balance or peace?

JOURNAL — My Notes

_____   _____
_____   _____
_____   _____
_____   _____
_____   _____
_____   _____
_____   _____
_____   _____

DAY 20
The spiral that holds center

旋中功
Traditional Name: Xuan Zhong Gong — "Spiraling from the Center"
Focus: To engage your core axis while your arms, legs and torso spiral around it, building dynamic balance: you move, but your center r

PREPARATION & BASE BREATHING
Sit or stand tall with feet grounded and spine gently lifted.
Inhale to widen the lower belly; exhale to let your center settle quietly.
Make small hip or ankle circles to awaken gentle rotation in the body.
Place hands on lower belly; inhale to expand, exhale to return to your calm axis.

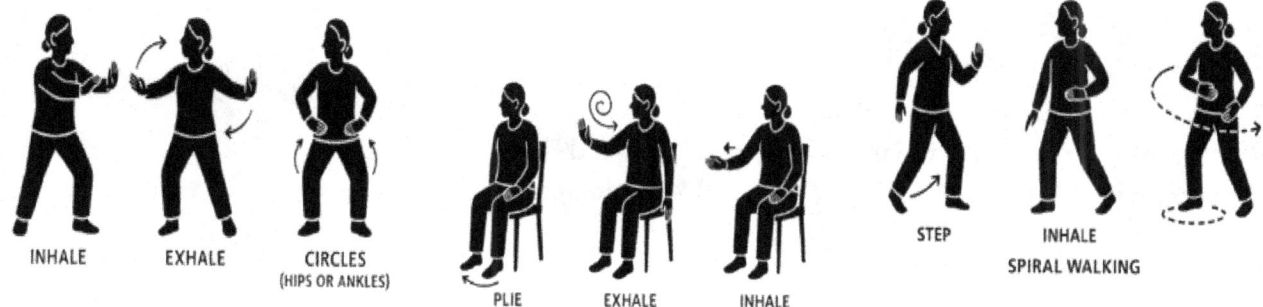

1-Torso twist and arm arc   2-Spiral Step   3-Flowing Spiral Walk

LEVEL 1 — Torso twist
Inhale to lengthen the spine; exhale to rotate softly right or left.
Let one arm sweep across the body as the torso follows in a small spiral.
Return to center on the inhale, alternating smooth spirals. 8 cycles

LEVEL 2 — Spiral Step- 8 cycles
Step diagonally forward as arms trace a soft outward spiral.
Exhale to complete the step; inhale to return to your center.
Alternate sides, keeping the movement fluid and initiated from your core.

LEVEL 3 — Flowing Spiral Walk- 8 cycles
Walk a short-curved path, letting torso and arms follow in gentle spirals.
Inhale to begin each step; exhale to land and settle your weight.
Move as if drawing a small spiral on the floor, stable yet fluid.

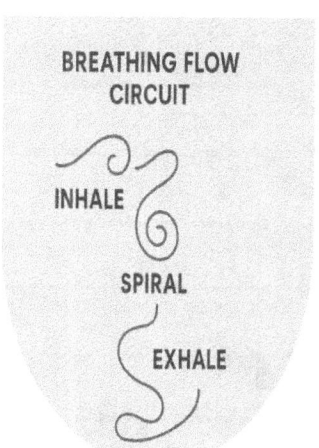

49

BODY & WELLBEING BENEFITS

AREA	BODY BENEFIT	DAILY EFFECT
Spine & Ribs	Improves rotational mobility	Easier turning & reaching behind you
Hips & Shoulders	Releases stiffness and tension	Freer movement in daily tasks
Whole Body	Coordinated spiral movement	Safer changes of direction

THERAPEUTIC TIPS
Move from the center, not the shoulders alone.
Keep spirals soft—avoid forcing range or speed.
Let exhalation guide the return toward your stable axis.

REFLECTION OF THE DAY

- Where did I feel the spiral most clearly—hips, ribs, shoulders or spine?
- Did my center stay quiet while my body moved outward?
- Where in my life could I allow a gentle "spiral"—a change without losing my stability?

JOURNAL — My Notes

DAY 21
The quiet center, the moving edge

静中动功
Traditional Name: Jing Zhong Dong Gong — "Stillness Within Movement"
Focus: To unite a calm inner center with gentle outer motion. You practice moving at your edges (arms, legs, steps) while your core remains steady and quietly present.

PREPARATION & BASE BREATHING
Sit or stand tall with feet grounded and knees soft.
Shift gently side-to-side to feel your weight settle.
Lift arms lightly on an inhale, lower on a soft exhale.
Hands on lower belly—inhale to expand, exhale to anchor.

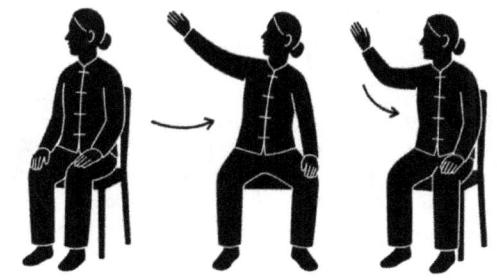
1-Edge Awareness

LEVEL 1 — Edge Awareness
Inhale at center, exhale as you reach slightly toward one side.
Return to center on the inhale, switching sides with ease.
Keep movements small, sensing the boundary of your reach. Repeat 8 cycles.

LEVEL 2 — Center–Edge Link
Step or slide one foot diagonally as the same-side arm extends.
Exhale to reach toward the "edge," inhale to return to center.
Repeat slowly, feeling your center support each outward motion. For 8 cycles

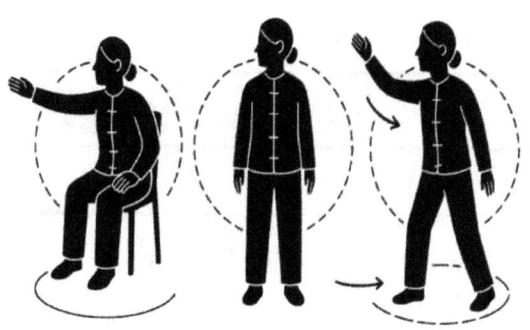
2-Center–Edge Link

LEVEL 3 — Expanding Edge Reach
Imagine a circle around you and choose points to reach toward.
Exhale as you step or slide toward a point; inhale to return home.
Explore 3–4 edges, moving calmly through your steady center.

3-Expanding Edge Reach

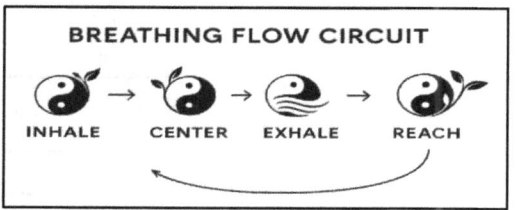

51

BODY & WELLBEING BENEFITS

AREA	BODY BENEFIT	DAILY EFFECT
Core & Hips	Strengthens center while limbs move	Safer reaching & side-stepping
Spine & Ribs	Improves rotational ease	Better turning & looking behind
Whole Body	Expands movement with stability	More confidence reaching outward

THERAPEUTIC TIPS
Allow movement at the edges, but keep breath soft at the center.
Keep steps and reaches small—exploration, not strain.
Return through center every time to train balance and orientation.

REFLECTION OF THE DAY

- When did my center feel the most steady today?
- Which "edge" felt easiest or most challenging to explore?
- Did I notice a moment where my movement and breath felt connected?

JOURNAL — My Notes

_____   _____
_____   _____
_____   _____
_____   _____
_____   _____
_____   _____
_____   _____

SPECIAL CONCLUSION TO WEEK 3: BALANCING

Harmony of Ground and Sky.

You've completed Week 3 of your journey—a week of exploring balance not as a static pose, but as a living process: one foot forward, one arm out, one breath more. You've trained your body and your mind to find stillness even as you move, and to move with awareness even as you're still.
Maybe you noticed a subtle shift: your step more confident, your reach more intentional, your posture more aware. Perhaps you recognized that the edge of your comfort zone isn't danger—it's growth.

Reflect now (and write if you like):

• Which day this week made you feel most balanced—calm inside, moving outside?
• When did you feel your centre anchor you even in motion?
• What kind of "edge" do you still feel drawn to explore—and how will you approach it with both strength and ease?

And if life got busy and you missed a movement or two: that's okay. Balance isn't about perfection—it's about returning, realigning, reconnecting. Every session, every breath, adds to your harmony.

Rest in this moment. Let your body and mind absorb what you've built. The path ahead is not about adding more—it's about deepening the meaning. Next week we'll continue onward, grounded, centred, moving with grace.
You are steady. You are open. You are balanced.

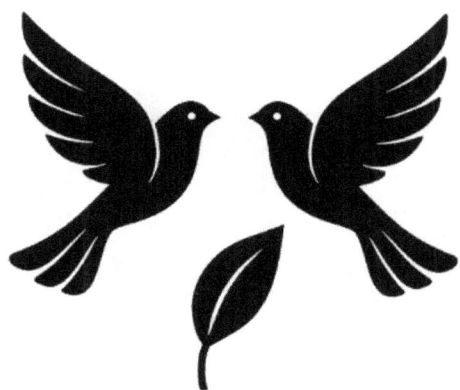

I invite you to reflect on

your first week

This is
your time
with
yourself

Dear Reader,

Thank you for being here and for giving yourself this time.

This book was created especially to support adults over 60 on a gentle path of movement, breathing, and reconnection with the body — honoring the rhythms, limits, and needs that naturally change over time.

But this journey does not end on these pages.

As part of this program, I have prepared a set of complementary resources designed to support this stage of life with care and kindness:

— Guided videos of the movements, with clear and unhurried explanations

— Guided meditation and relaxation audio to calm the nervous system

— A quick guide for days when the body asks for extra gentleness

— Short practices to restore balance and presence

— Therapeutic mandalas for moments of calm and focus

— Soft music to accompany practice, rest, or reading

— And a 28-day calendar to gently support your process

These materials are not another demand or rigid program.

They are a supportive space so you can adapt the practice to your body, your daily energy, and your own rhythm.

To access them, you may:

• **Scan the QR code included with this book.**

No video downloads are required.

Watch it instantly and practice anytime, on any device.

If you wish, you can have the PDF materials in print; they are enabled for one-click printing.

My intention is simply to walk alongside you —

supporting calm, stability, and confidence in your body,

one gentle step at a time.

Thank you for walking this path with me.

With care,

Fabiana Renacer

Your bonuses are here

And now, we gently continue…

**As you enter the final week of this practice,
allow yourself to move with even more kindness,
listening closely to what your body needs each day.**

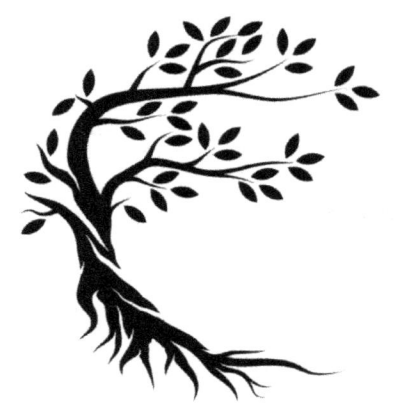

CHAPTER 6 -WEEK 4- Flow
Day 22-The stream of movement

流水功

Traditional Name: Liú Shuǐ Gōng — "Flowing Water Practice"

Focus: To move continuously and naturally, like water flowing around stones. You integrate strength, balance, and breath into soft, fluid transitions.

PREPARATION & BASE BREATHING
Sit or stand tall with feet grounded and knees soft.
Lift arms gently on the inhale, lower them softly on the exhale.
Sway slightly side to side, letting movement feel round and continuous.
Hands on lower belly—inhale to expand, exhale to let tension flow downward.

LEVEL 1 — Shoulder & Spine Circles- 8 cycles
Inhale as arms lift; exhale as they open.
Roll shoulders in soft circles, letting the upper spine follow.
Repeat slowly, keeping the movement fluid and relaxed.

LEVEL 2 — Flow Step- 8 cycles
Slide one foot forward as the opposite arm rises in a soft arc.
Exhale to return smoothly to center, switching sides with ease.
Let each step pour into the next without sharp edges or pauses.

LEVEL 3 — Continuous Water Sequence
Step gently forward while arms open and torso turns slightly.
Exhale to return to center in one smooth, connected motion.
Flow through 5–6 steps, creating a seamless stream of movement.

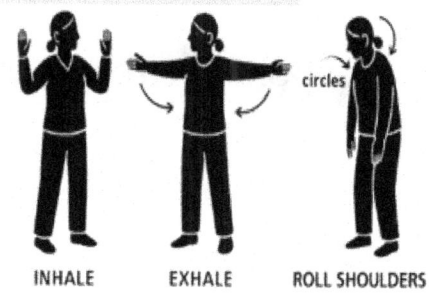

1-Shoulder and spine circles

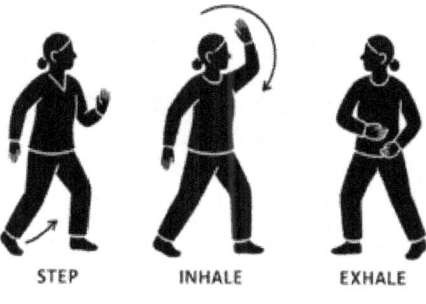

2-Flow Step

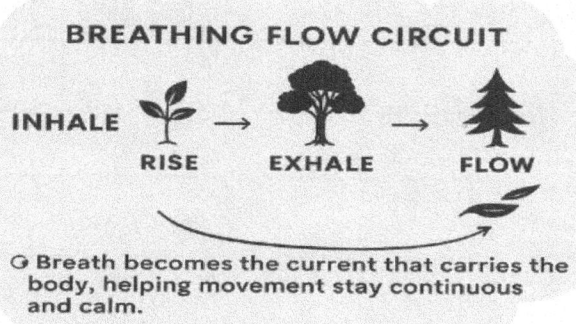

Breath becomes the current that carries the body, helping movement stay continuous and calm.

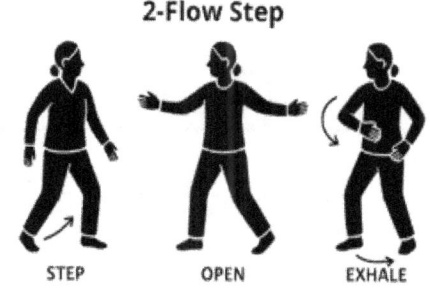

3-Continuous Sequence

BODY & WELLBEING BENEFITS

AREA	BODY BENEFIT	DAILY EFFECT
Spine & Ribs	Improved body rotation	Easier turning & reaching
Hips & Feet	Smooth directional changes	Safer stepping & transitions
Whole Body	Coordination & fluidity	Less stiffness, more grace in motions

THERAPEUTIC TIPS
Let the breath be the "current" that moves the body.
Replace sharp movements with curves and spirals.
Imagine your body adapting like water moving around a stone.

REFLECTION OF THE DAY

- What part of today's practice felt most fluid or natural?
- How did it feel to move without pausing—strange, freeing, calming?
- Where in your life could more "flow" lighten your movement or decisions?

JOURNAL — My Notes

DAY 23
The wave of continuity

震流功
Traditional Name: Zhen Liu Gong — "Practice of Perpetual Flow"
Focus: To let movement flow without stops or stiffness. Like waves rolling one after another, you connect breath, arms, core and legs in a smooth, continuous rhythm.

PREPARATION & BASE BREATHING
Sit or stand tall with feet grounded and knees soft.
Lift arms gently on the inhale, lower them softly on the exhale.
Shift your weight lightly side to side to awaken your base.
Place hands on lower belly; inhale to expand, exhale to settle.

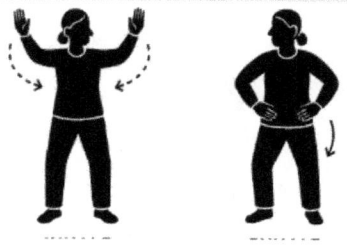

1-Gentle Wave Motion

LEVEL 1 — Gentle Wave Motion- 8 cycles
Inhale to lengthen spine and lift arms softly.
Exhale to let arms flow outward and down like a small wave.
Return smoothly to center, keeping shoulders relaxed.

LEVEL 2 — Side Wave Step- 8 cycles
Step or slide one foot outward as arms follow in a gentle side wave.
Exhale as you travel toward the edge; inhale to return to center.
Alternate sides, keeping movement continuous and soft.

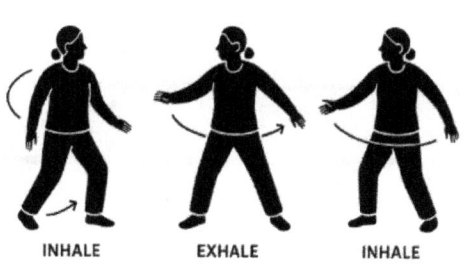

2-Linked Wave Chain

LEVEL 3 — Linked Wave Chain
Begin a small forward wave, then glide into a side wave without pausing.
Let breath guide each direction change—forward, then sideways.
Return to center smoothly, linking 4–5 flowing chains per side.

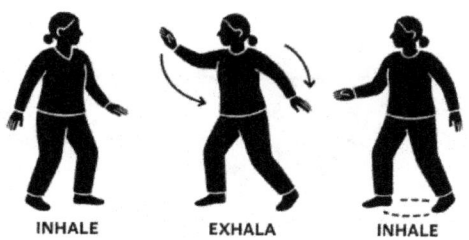

3-My movement flows

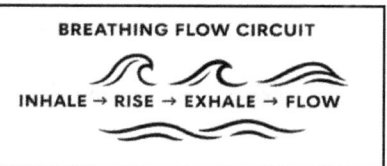

BODY & WELLBEING BENEFITS

AREA	BODY BENEFIT	DAILY EFFECT
Spine & Ribs	Smoother wave motion	Easier turning & reaching
Hips & Legs	Fluid weight shifts	Softer steps & direction changes
Whole Body	Continuous coordination	Less stiffness & fewer stops

Therapeutic Tips
Let breath set the rhythm—never force the wave. Keep knees soft so the body can "roll" with ease. Imagine water moving around obstacles rather than pushing through them.

REFLECTION OF THE DAY

- Where did I feel the wave most clearly in my body?
- Was it easy or challenging to keep movement continuous?
- Where in my life could more flow help things move with ease?

JOURNAL — My Notes

DAY 24
The river of rhythm

和流功

Traditional Name: He Liu Gong — "Harmony in Flow"
Focus: To move in rhythm with your breath and body. Today you practice transitions, linking movements together in a steady current so that motion feels both effortless and intentional.

PREPARATION & BASE BREATHING
Sit or stand with feet grounded and knees soft.
Let arms rest and gently close your eyes.
Inhale like a calm stream filling your center; exhale to soften and release tension.
Imagine your body moving like water—adapting, curving, and continuing with ease.

LEVEL 1 — Rhythm Reach
Inhale to lift both arms forward to chest height.
Exhale to sweep them down in a soft arc, adding a tiny knee bend or lean.
Return to center smoothly, keeping breath and motion in one rhythm. Repeat 8 cycles.

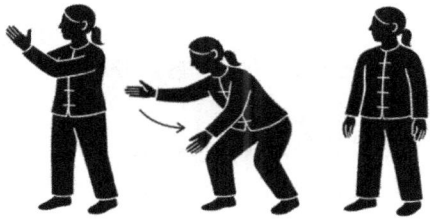

LEVEL 2 — Flow Step & Reach. 8 cycles
Step slightly forward or to the side as your arms trace a gentle arc.
Exhale into the reach; inhale to return to center.
Alternate sides for smooth, breath-led transitions.

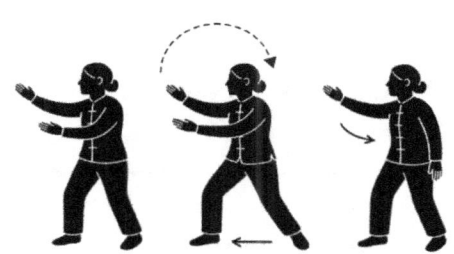

LEVEL 3 — Continuous River Sequence- 8 cycles
Step outward, let arms wave up, and add a comfortable torso rotation.
Exhale to return to center in one unbroken motion.
Repeat small flowing cycles, like water curving around stones.

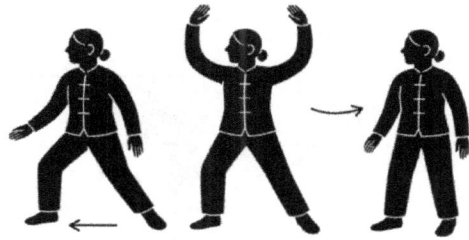

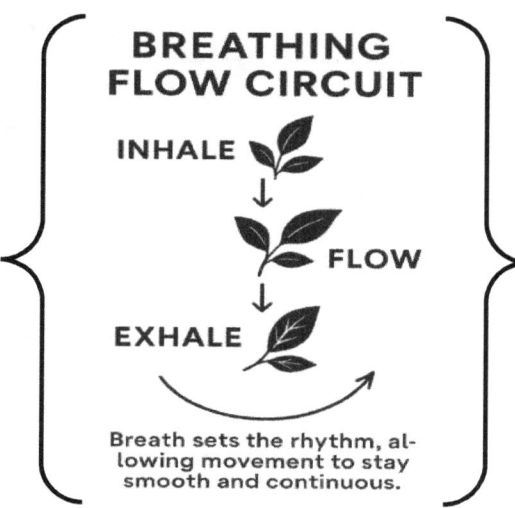

BODY & WELLBEING BENEFITS

AREA	BODY BENEFIT	DAILY EFFECT
Spine & Ribs	Enhances rhythmic mobility	Smoother turning & reaching
Hips & Legs	Supports flowing steps	Softer transitions & direction change
Whole Body	Builds continuous movement	Less stiffness, fewer pauses

THERAPEUTIC TIPS
Move as if avoiding sharp edges—round, gentle, uninterrupted.
Keep steps small so rhythm stays soft and steady.
Let the exhale guide each fluid transition.

REFLECTION OF THE DAY

- How did it feel to move in rhythm instead of stop-and-start?
- What moment felt most fluid or natural?
- Where in my life could more "flow" ease tension or resistance?

JOURNAL — My Notes

_____   _____
_____   _____
_____   _____
_____   _____
_____   _____
_____   _____
_____   _____

DIA 25
The circle of breath and movement

循环气功

Traditional Name: Xun Qi Gong — "Circulation of Breath Practice"
Focus: To bring your breath and motion into a gentle loop — moving in circles and arcs so your body, energy, and awareness flow in one smooth cycle.

PREPARATION & BASE BREATHING
Sit or stand tall with feet grounded and knees soft.
Inhale: imagine a soft circle of light expanding from your lower belly.
Exhale: feel the circle travel up, around your torso, and back to center.
Repeat 3 slow breaths, tracing this inner loop with ease.

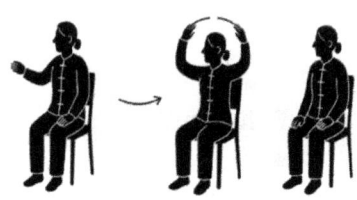
LEVEL 1 – Simple Circle Reach

LEVEL 1 — Simple Circle Reach
Inhale to lift arms forward; exhale to draw a wide, smooth circle overhead.
Let the circle stay soft and continuous, with relaxed shoulders.
Return to center through the same calm loop. For 8 cycles.

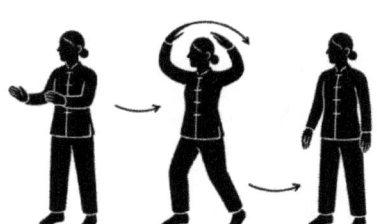
LEVEL 2 – Circle Step & Reach

LEVEL 2 — Circle Step & Reach- 8 cycles
Step gently to the side as your arms draw a full overhead circle.
Let inhale prepare you; exhale guides the step and circle together.
Return to center and alternate sides in one coordinated motion.

LEVEL 3 — Flowing Spiral Cycle - 8 cycles
Step diagonally forward while circling the arms in a wide loop.
Allow a gentle torso rotation before returning smoothly to center.
Each finished circle becomes the beginning of the next spiral.

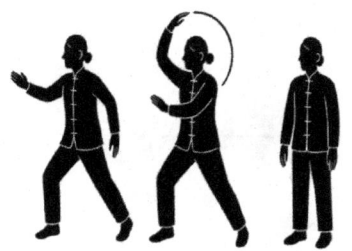
LEVEL 3 – Flowing Spiral Cycle

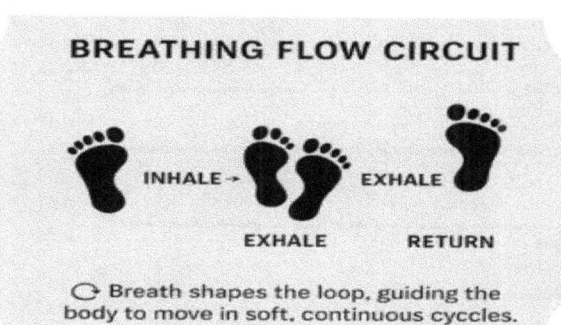
BREATHING FLOW CIRCUIT
INHALE → EXHALE
EXHALE   RETURN
↻ Breath shapes the loop, guiding the body to move in soft, continuous cycles.

BODY & WELLBEING BENEFITS

AREA	BODY BENEFIT	DAILY EFFECT
Shoulders & Spine	Encourages circular mobility	Freer turning & reaching
Hips & Legs	Supports coordinated stepping	Smoother directional changes
Whole Body	Builds rhythmic connection	Less stiffness, more flow

THERAPEUTIC TIPS
Let breath set the size of each circle—never force the motion.
Keep circles soft and round, like drawing with air.
Always return through your center before beginning the next loop.

REFLECTION OF THE DAY

- Where did I feel the circle most clearly today—arms, ribs, hips?
- Was it natural or new to keep the movement continuous?
- What simple cycle in my daily life could benefit from this "circle → return" rhythm?

JOURNAL — My Notes

DAY 26
The breath that carries motion

气带动功

Traditional Name: Qi Dai Dong Gong — "Breath-Driven Motion Practice"
Focus: To align your breath with your body's motion so that each movement becomes an expression of your inner rhythm. Today you practice flowing through action and breath as one seamless experience

PREPARATION & BASE BREATHING
Sit or stand tall, feet grounded and knees soft.
Inhale slowly through the nose, exhale softly through the mouth.
Let breath feel like a gentle wind preparing your body to move.
Hands on lower belly: inhale to expand, exhale to soften.

LEVEL 1 — Breath-Wave Reach- 8 cycles
Inhale to lift arms forward and up to a comfortable height.
Exhale to sweep arms down and slightly behind the body.
Repeat smoothly, letting breath set the rhythm.

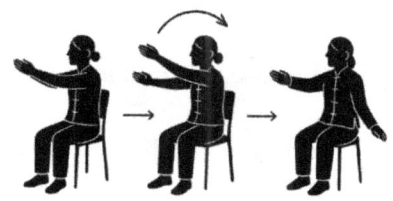
Level 1-Breath wave reach

LEVEL 2 — Step with Breath Carry - 8 cycles
Inhale at center to prepare.
Exhale to step lightly forward as arms follow a natural walking motion.
Inhale to return; switch sides with calm, steady timing.

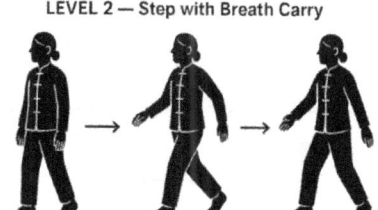
LEVEL 2 — Step with Breath Carry

LEVEL 3 — Full Breath Flow Sequence - 8 cycles
Inhale to lengthen spine and prepare.
Exhale to step forward, lift arms, and add a soft torso turn toward the stepping side.
Inhale to return to center; repeat in a slow alternating flow.

LEVEL 3 — Full Breath Flow Sequence
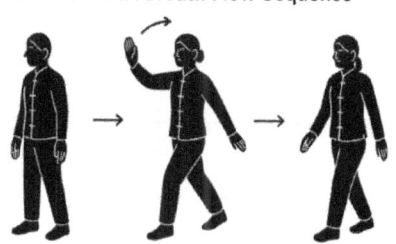

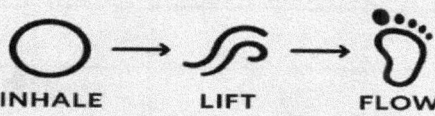

BODY & WELLBEING BENEFITS

AREA	BODY BENEFIT	DAILY EFFECT
Chest & Ribs	Expands breathing space	Deeper, calmer breath
Core	Activates naturally	Safer, smoother steps
Whole Body	Syncs motion to breath	Less tension & rushing

THERAPEUTIC TIPS
Let breath be the "conductor" of each movement.
Keep steps small and smooth.
Exhale into motion; inhale back to center.

REFLECTION OF THE DAY

- When did you most clearly feel that your breath was guiding your movement?

- Where did your rhythm become uncoordinated… and what changed when you slowed down?

- In what area of your life would you like to "breathe first, act later"?

JOURNAL — My Notes

_____   _____
_____   _____
_____   _____
_____   _____
_____   _____
_____   _____

DAY 27
The full current within

全流功

Traditional Name: Quan Liu Gong — "Whole-Flow Practice"

Focus: To experience your practice as one continuous current of movement—from your feet or hips to your arms and breath—combining everything you've learned into a single, integrated flow.

PREPARATION & BASE BREATHING
Sit or stand tall with feet grounded and knees soft.
Inhale to feel breath rise through your center.
Exhale to let your weight settle into the floor or chair.
Repeat 3 breaths, sensing a gentle current beginning inside you.

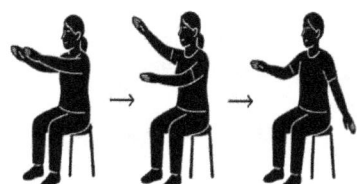

LEVEL 1 — Current Initiation - 8 cycles
Inhale to lift both arms forward with a soft rise.
Exhale to lower arms as feet or sitting bones gently ground.
Repeat slow waves, letting movement start from your center.

LEVEL 2 — Flow Link - 8 cycles
Step slightly forward or sideways as arms circle outward and up.
Inhale to begin the circle; exhale to settle and return.
Let legs power the circle so the whole body moves as one.

LEVEL 3 — Whole-Body Flow Run - 8 cycles
Step and circle your arms while adding a gentle torso turn.
Exhale to complete the sequence; inhale to reset at center.
Link cycles smoothly, like one uninterrupted current.

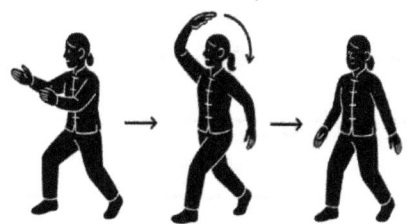

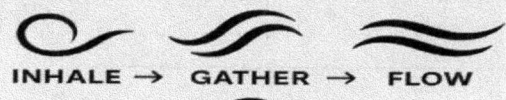

BREATHING FLOW CIRCUIT

INHALE → GATHER → FLOW

Breath unifies the body, guiding one continuous current from step to step.

BODY & WELLBEING BENEFITS

AREA	BODY BENEFIT	DAILY EFFECT
Core & Breath.	Unifies upper & lower body	Smoother walking & turning
Legs & Feet	Strengthens grounding	Safer steps, less wobbling
Whole Body	Builds continuous flow	Less stiffness, fewer stop-points

THERAPEUTIC TIPS
Let breath set the timing of each move.
Keep steps small and circles smooth.
Imagine the whole body moving like one soft current.

REFLECTION OF THE DAY

- Where did I feel the current most clearly in my body today?
- Which transition felt the most fluid… or the most interrupted?
- In which daily action would I like to apply more "whole-flow"?

JOURNAL — My Notes

_____   _____
_____   _____
_____   _____
_____   _____
_____   _____
_____   _____
_____   _____

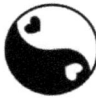

DAY 28

The flow that carries forever

永流功

Traditional Name: *Yong Liu Gong* — "Practice of Eternal Flow"
Focus: To celebrate what you've built in these 4 weeks—strength, balance, and fluidity—and feel your whole body moving as one continuous current. This day is both an ending and a new beginning.

> **PREPARATION & BASE BREATHING**
> Sit or stand tall with feet grounded and knees soft.
> Inhale to open the chest; exhale to settle your weight.
> Shift gently side to side, sensing a calm base.
> Hands on lower belly: inhale to expand, exhale to gather your flow inward.

LEVEL 1 — Gentle Continuum - 8 cycles
Inhale to lift arms forward to chest height.
Exhale to open arms outward and relax them down.
Feel a smooth wave from center to fingertips.

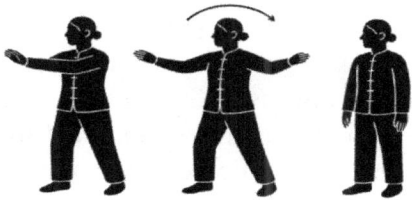
LEVEL 1 – Gentle Continuum

LEVEL 2 — Flow Step & Arms - 8 cycles
Step one foot forward or sideways with the inhale.
Exhale as arms rise and float back while returning to center.
Alternate sides in one steady rhythm.

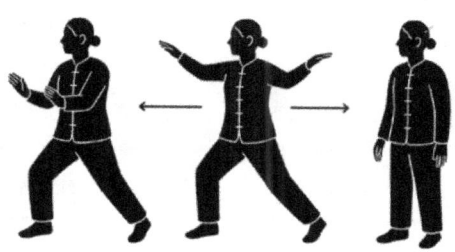
LEVEL 2 – Flow Step & Arms

LEVEL 3 — Complete Flow Cycle - 8 cycles
Step forward or sideways and let arms arc upward.
Add a soft torso turn toward the stepping side.
Return to center smoothly, letting each cycle flow into the next.

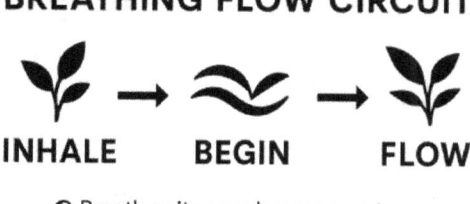

BREATHING FLOW CIRCUIT
INHALE → BEGIN → FLOW
↩ Breath unites each movement, completing the cycle with calm continuity.

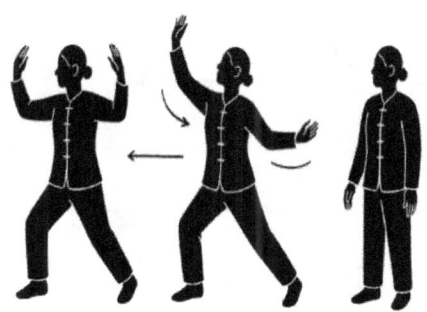
LEVEL 3 – Complete Flow Cycle

BODY & WELLBEING BENEFITS

AREA	BODY BENEFIT	DAILY EFFECT
Whole Body	Coordinates full-body flow	Walking & turning feel smoother
Core & Breath	Strengthens center-led movement	More stability with less effort
Mind–Body	Connects motion into one rhythm	Promotes calm, confidence & ease

THERAPEUTIC TIPS
Let breath set the tempo—movement follows.
Keep steps small and gentle to maintain continuity.
Imagine each cycle finishing exactly where the next begins.

REFLECTION OF THE DAY

- Which part of my body felt this "continuous flow" most clearly?
- Were there moments of complete softness… or interruptions?
- In which daily action do I want to bring this sense of continuity?

JOURNAL — My Notes

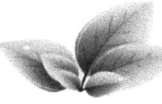

I invite you to reflect on

your first week

- Where did I feel the most flow this week?

- What movement felt smooth… or interrupted?

- Where in daily life do I want more flow?

This is your time with yourself

SPECIAL CLOSING · COMPLETING THE 28-DAY JOURNEY

A New Beginning in Motion

You have completed the 28-day program — **but this is not the end**.
Your body now moves with more awareness, softness and unity.
You strengthened your base, awakened your breath, trained balance, and learned to flow.

This final week taught you to **connect everything** into one living rhythm.

Bonus Material — Your Next Step

These resources deepen your practice by offering:
- Extra mini-routines for busy days
- Gentle adaptations for low-energy days
- Reflections that support emotional and physical clarity
- Movement variations to grow your confidence even more

They help you **maintain your progress** instead of losing it.

Don't Skip the Next Chapters

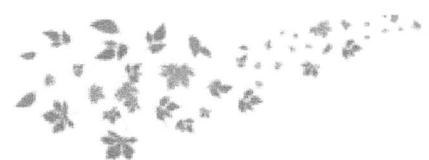

They will guide you to:
- Understand why these movements calm your body
- Adjust the practice to your real-life rhythm
- Turn this 28-day routine into a simple daily ritual

Move through them slowly. Let every insight become part of your day.

Your Practice Can Continue in Many Ways

You may choose to:
- Repeat the journey at a deeper level
- Create a short daily flow
- Teach movements to someone you love
- Use the bonus practices as a weekly cycle

Each repetition takes you **forward**, not back.

Stay Curious

New books in this series will bring:
• Flows for memory, rest, confidence, focus
• Emotional resilience practices
• More Tai Chi–inspired sequences for everyday life

Ask yourself gently:
"How else could my body and life feel… if I continue just a little more?"

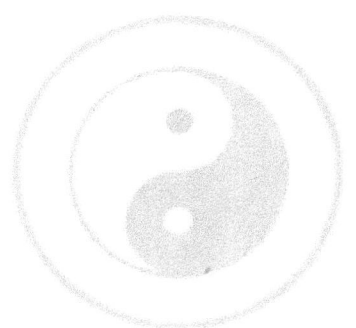

THANK YOU FOR SHOWING UP — DAY AFTER DAY

You are steadier.
You are softer.
You are stronger.
You flow — and this is only the beginning.

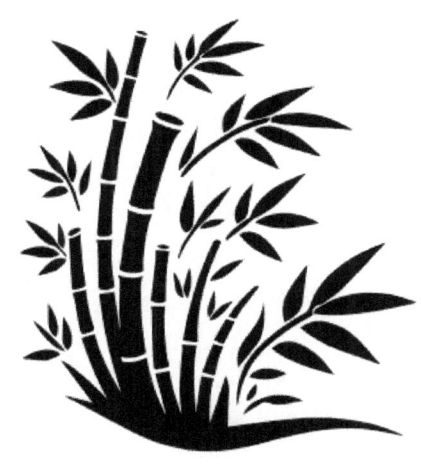

"IT'S NEVER TOO LATE TO START OVER"

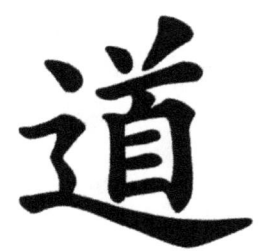

CHAPTER 7
Tai Chi for Memory, Mood & Emotional Well-Being

Tai Chi is not only movement for the body.
It is also one of the simplest ways to keep the mind awake, steady, and emotionally balanced as we age.
Many people over 60 notice that after just a few days of gentle practice, they feel clearer, calmer, and more present.
This is not magic—it is how the brain responds to slow, coordinated movement, breath, and mindful attention.
This chapter explains, in simple terms, **why Tai Chi is so good for your mind**, and how you can use it to support memory, mood, and emotional health every day.

Tai Chi and the Brain: Focus, Memory & Attention

Tai Chi stimulates the brain in a unique way:
you move slowly enough for the brain to *notice* every shift, every breath, every transition.
This creates a kind of "mental training" that feels gentle but reaches deep.

Research shows that Tai Chi can help improve:

- **Focus and attention** — because slow movement requires presence.
- **Memory and recall** — because you repeat patterns and coordinate arms, legs, and breath.
- **Processing speed** — the brain becomes more efficient at organizing movement.
- **Mind–body connection** — awareness grows with each practice.

For older adults, this kind of training is protective.
It keeps the brain active without overwhelming it.

The goal is not perfection.
The goal is **engagement**—keeping your mind gently awake inside your movements.

Slow Movement Against Stress & Anxiety

Stress and anxiety don't go away with age—sometimes they increase.
Tai Chi offers something that most forms of exercise do not:

It teaches the body how to calm down while still moving.
When you move slowly and breathe deeply:

- Your **nervous system shifts from stress mode to relaxation mode**.
- Your heart rate lowers naturally.

- Muscle tension releases.
- The mind becomes quieter without forcing anything.

Many people describe Tai Chi as "moving meditation" because the body becomes busy while the mind becomes peaceful.

This calm isn't fragile.
It begins to follow you into daily life:

- When you're getting up from a chair
- When you're walking through a crowded aisle
- When you're dealing with a difficult moment

Tai Chi builds emotional resilience through softness, not pressure.

Moving Meditation: The Power of Breathing While You Walk

One of the most accessible forms of Tai Chi is something we already do every day: **walking**.

When you coordinate your steps with your breath:

- The mind stops jumping from thought to thought.
- The body feels more grounded and secure.
- Worries lose intensity.
- A sense of presence grows naturally.

Try this simple practice:

1. **Inhale for one step.**
2. **Exhale for the next two steps.**
3. Walk slowly and let your arms swing naturally.
4. Keep your eyes soft, looking a few feet ahead.

This "walking breath" is a powerful emotional tool.
It brings peace without needing a mat, a chair, or a special setup.

You can use it:

- In the morning to start calmly.
- In the evening to release the day.
- Anytime you feel overwhelmed.

It becomes a gentle companion for daily life.

Why This Matters After 60

With age, we need movement that supports *the whole person*.
Tai Chi does exactly that:

- It **protects the brain**.
- It **calms the heart and the emotions**.
- It **reduces fear**, especially the fear of falling.
- It **creates a feeling of confidence** from the inside out.

Many older adults say:

"I feel more like myself again."

Not because they move faster, but because they move with **clarity, calm, and trust**.

A Gentle Reminder

You don't need to do long sessions to get these benefits.
Even **5–10 minutes a day** of slow movement and intentional breathing can bring:

- A clearer mind
- A lighter mood
- A more grounded emotional state

The more consistently you practice, the more these effects accumulate—quietly, steadily, and reliably.

Inner Reflection

You may take a moment to write:

- When did my mind feel clearest during practice this week?
- Did the slow movements help me calm down?
- Where in my life could I use more "moving calm"?

A few lines are enough.
They help you see how Tai Chi supports not only your body, but your whole inner life.

CHAPTER 8
Adaptations for common conditions

Practical, safe, natural ways to adjust Tai Chi to your body.

OSTEOPOROSIS			
What Happens	What Helps	Avoid	Safe Adjustments
Reduced bone density, fear of falling.	Small weight shifts chair, support; slow arcs.	Sudden twists, deep bends.	Movements small; feet grounded; light hand on chair.

VERTIGO			
What Happens	What Helps	Avoid	Safe Adjustments
Spinning sensation; insecurity shifting weight.	Fixed gaze; seated arc; slow transitions.	Quick head turns, fast stepping.	Minimize rotation; start seated; eyes on one point.

ARTHRITIS / ARTHROSIS			
What Happens	What Helps	Avoid	Safe Adjustments
Stiff joints, reduced range.	Circular motions, gentle arcs.	Forced range, deep bends.	Knees soft; circles small, relaxed pace.

CHRONIC FATIGUE			
What Happens	What Helps	Avoid	Safe Adjustments
Quick fatigue; low stamina.	Seated practice. breath-led arms.	Long routines; fast pace.	Short sessions; micro-steps. focus on exhale.

How to Use This Chapter:
Find your condition → Choose the safe adjustment → Follow the adaptation route → Apply to your 28-day practice.

KNEE PAIN

What Happens	What Helps	Avoid	Safe Adjustments
Pain with bending-stepping.	Hip-led movement; small steps.	Twisting on knee; deep bends.	Knees aligned with toes; shorter stance; chair nearby.

BALANCE INSECURITY

What Happens	What Helps	Avoid	Safe Adjustments
Fear of falling; stiffness when stepping.	Chair support; wide stance; slow shifts.	Narrow stance; fast transitions.	Eyes forward; calm pace; feet hip-width.

TAI CHI WITH CHAIR

Ideal For	Benefits	Key Adjustments
Vertigo, fatigue, early practice days.	Zero fall risk, full breath training.	Sit on edge; spine long; arms free.

How to Use This Chapter:
Find your condition → Choose the safe adjustment → Follow the adaptation route → Apply to your 28-day practice.

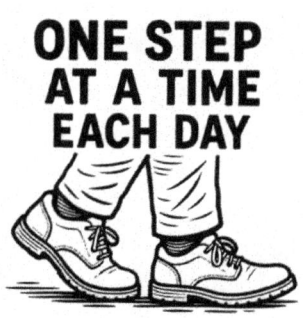

CHAPTER 9
What Happens After the 28 Days? Your Path Forward

You've completed the 28-day journey—an achievement many people intend to begin but never finish. And now a natural question appears:

"What do I do next?"

The answer is simple and encouraging:
You keep going, but in a way that feels sustainable, personal, and enjoyable for your life.
This chapter gives you a gentle roadmap, so your progress doesn't fade, but becomes a new foundation for how you move, breathe, and live.

Repeat the Cycle—With New Awareness

Your body learns through repetition.
When you repeat this 28-day program, you don't return to the beginning—you return **higher**, with more balance, more confidence, and more connection.
Many older adults notice on the second round:
- The movements feel smoother.
- Breath and body sync more naturally.
- Strength shows up in small, everyday actions.
- Fear of falling begins to soften.

You can repeat the full cycle or choose only one week at a time:
- **Week 1** if you need grounding and calm.
- **Week 2** if you want more strength and stability.
- **Week 3** if you feel stiff and want space and mobility.
- **Week 4** if you crave flow and rhythm.

Let your needs guide the choice.

Build Your Own Short Routine

(Your Personal 5–10 Minute Practice)

After the program, many people prefer a **simple daily "maintenance flow."**
You can create yours by choosing:
- **1 preparation breath routine**
- **1 main movement** (your favorite from any day)
- **1 cool-down**
- **1 affirmation**

This takes **5 minutes** yet keeps the benefits alive.

A few examples:

For balance days:
- Preparation breath + Level 2 weight shift + gentle torso turn + "I move with steady confidence."

For stiff-back days:
- Seated breath + circle arms + side wave + "I create space inside me."

For anxious days:
- Inhale 4/exhale 6 + slow arm sweep + seated version of any movement + "I soften into this moment."

Tiny routines create long-term change.

Practice With Others

(If You Want To—No Pressure)

Tai Chi grows beautifully in community.
You may explore:
- A local senior center offering gentle movement classes
- A Tai Chi group at a park
- Online videos for older adults
- Practicing with a friend or partner at home

Practicing with others can increase motivation and joy—but it is completely optional.
Your body is already your best teacher.

Helpful Resources to Support You

Your journey continues beyond this book. You now have:
- **Your Inner Journey Notebook** → to track small victories
- **Your favorite movements** → to repeat anytime
- **All three levels** → to adapt to your daily energy
- **Calming micro-practices** → for stress, pain, or sleepless nights
- **Simple breathwork tools** → that travel with you everywhere

Each of these tools is designed to stay with you for months and years, not just 28 days.

A Daily Ritual That Keeps You Growing

If you choose just **one practice** to continue, let it be this:

Pause. Breathe. Move slowly for one minute.

Even a single mindful minute:
- Improves balance
- Calms your nervous system
- Reduces stiffness
- Increases awareness
- Strengthens your connection with your body

This one-minute ritual is your long-term anchor.

Final Message: You Are in Motion Now

Finishing 28 days is not the end—it's the doorway.

You now know:
- How to listen to your body
- How to choose your level
- How to move without fear
- How to breathe through challenge
- How to reconnect with your own inner flow

Your next steps don't have to be big.
One gentle step each day is enough.
Carry this quiet truth forward:
"My practice continues—not because I must, but because it helps me live better."

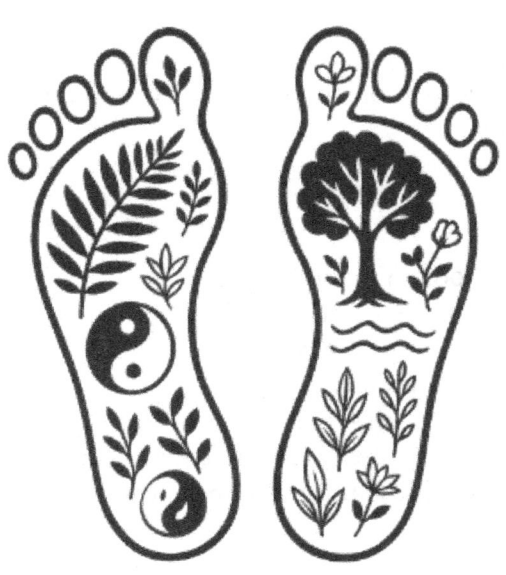

"LITTLE STEPS MATTER"

TAI CHI ESSENTIAL GLOSSARY

A gentle guide to the words you'll meet in this book

氣 —Qi (Energy Vitality)	Natural life force that animates the body. When it flows freely, movement feels light and calm.
丹田 —Dantian (Energy Center)	Located below the navel, your internal base. All balanced movement begins and returns here.
鬆 —Song (Release / Softening)	Letting go of tension without collapsing. Creates relaxed strength and smoother movement.
勁 —Peng (Soft Expansive Strength)	Gentle, buoyant internal support. Builds upright posture without stiffness or force.
根 —Rooting (Grounding Stability)	Feeling steady through feet or sitting bones. Essential for safe walking, stepping, and turning.
樁 —Zhan Zhuang (Standing Stillness)	Quiet standing posture developing inner strength. Trains calm focus and whole-body alignment.
氣息 —Mindful Breath	Breath guides movement rather than chasing it. Inhale prepares; exhale carries you into motion.
轉換 —Weight Shift	Gentle transfer of weight side-to-side. Improves balance, leg strength, and walking confidence.
螺旋 —Spiral Movement	Soft turning through waist and ribs. Reduces stiffness and creates natural, fluid coordination.
圓 — Circular Motion	Moving in curves rather than straight lines. Protects joints and keeps transitions smooth.
坐太極 —Seated Tai Chi	Full Tai Chi benefits practiced from a chair. Supports safety while maintaining mind–body focus.
陰陽 —Yin–Yang (Balance of Opposites)	Harmony between effort and ease, stability and movement. Balance comes from listening, not forcing.

28-DAY TAI CHI PROGRAM- SUMMARY TABLE

Day	Theme / Main Focus	Core Benefit
1	Awakening the Breath	Calm activation, body awareness.
2	Grounding Through the Feet	Stable base, safer stepping.
3	Gentle Weight Shifts	Balance re-training.
4	Expanding the Chest	Easier breathing, posture.
5	Side-Body Mobility	Soft flexibility, torso ease.
6	Forward–Back Balance	Confidence in daily transitions.
7	Coordinated Arm Flow	Upper-body mobility, rhythm.
8	Leg Strength, Soft Activation	Stronger support without strain.
9	Hip-Friendly Shifts	Smoother walking pattern.
10	Diagonal Weight Transfer	Everyday turning made safer.
11	Step + Reach Patterns	Whole-body coordination.
12	Gentle Standing Strength	Upright stability, joint protection.
13	Core Engagement (Soft)	Safer posture, reduced fatigue.
14	Controlled Transitions	Confidence rising from chair & steps.
15	Circling Stillness	Smooth directional changes.
16	Moving Around Your Axis	Stable rotation, fall-prevention.
17	Building the Inner Bridge	Feet–core–arms connection.
18	Lightness & Weight	Balance between lifting and settling.
19	Rooting Into the Ground	Deeper stability, grounded steps.
20	Spiral Motion	Healthy spine, fluid turning.
21	Center & Edge Awareness	Move outward without losing balance.
22	Flowing Like Water	Continuous transitions, less stiffness.
23	Linked Wave Movements	Improved rhythm and endurance.
24	Rhythmic Movement	Natural timing, coordinated flow.
25	Circular Motion	Joint-friendly strength, mobility.
26	Breath-Led Movement	Breath guides action, calm stability.
27	Whole-Body Current	Unified movement, confidence.
28	Completing the Flow	Integration, readiness to continue.

REFERENCES – Trusted, Evidence-Based Sources

Medical & Scientific Organizations

- **Harvard Health Publishing** – Research on Tai Chi for balance, fall prevention, joint health, and emotional wellbeing.
- **Mayo Clinic** – Mind–body exercise benefits for aging, mobility, and chronic conditions.
- **National Institute on Aging (NIA)** – Guidelines for safe movement, strength, and balance for older adults.
- **Centers for Disease Control and Prevention (CDC)** – Fall-prevention strategies and physical activity recommendations.
- **World Health Organization (WHO)** – Healthy Aging principles and functional movement recommendations.
- **National Institutes of Health (NIH)** – Mind–body interventions and their effects on cognition, anxiety, and overall vitality.

TAI CHI & QIGONG – General Foundations

Traditional Styles (Non-Proprietary)

- **Yang Style Tai Chi** – Known for slow, expansive, gentle movements ideal for beginners and older adults.
- **Sun Style Tai Chi** – Features upright posture and smooth, flowing steps; excellent for joint protection.
- **Chen Style Tai Chi** – Rooted, spiraling movements with strong focus on core stability and coordination.

Universal Qigong Principles

- **Dantian Breathing (Lower-Belly Breath):**
  Supports balance, calmness, and core activation.
- **Rooting into the Ground:**
  Strengthens stability and teaches safe weight shifting.
- **Fluid, Continuous Motion:**
  Improves joint lubrication, circulation, and whole-body coordination.
- **Mindful Awareness:**
  Soft focus that reduces anxiety and supports cognitive clarity.

FAQ – Frequently Asked Questions

1. Do I need prior experience to start this program?

No. This 28-day journey is designed for complete beginners. Each day includes seated options and gentle levels so you can begin safely at any stage.

2. What if I have limited mobility or use a chair most of the day?

You can complete the entire program **seated** and still receive major benefits: better breathing, posture, mobility, awareness, and emotional calm.

3. What if I feel dizzy or unsteady sometimes?

Always choose **Level 1 or Level 2** and keep a chair nearby for support. Tai Chi's slow shifts improve stability gradually and safely.

4. Can I practice with osteoporosis, arthritis, or joint pain?

Yes—gently. This book includes specific adaptations. Slow, low-impact motion improves joint lubrication, strength, and balance without strain.

5. What if I miss a day?

Nothing is lost. Simply continue with the next day, or repeat the previous one if you want to deepen it. Consistency matters more than perfection.

6. Is Tai Chi enough as my main exercise?

For many adults 60+, Tai Chi can be a complete movement practice—improving strength, balance, mobility, breath, and mental health.

7. How long until I feel improvements?

Most people feel changes within **7–10 days**: easier walking, better balance, calmer breath, and less stiffness.

8. Can I continue the program once I finish the 28 days?

Yes. You can:
- repeat the whole journey,
- combine your favorite days into short routines,
- or follow the continuation ideas in Chapter 9.

9. Is it normal to wobble?

Absolutely. A wobble is not a failure—it's your body learning. Stability improves through gentle repetition.

10. What if I feel emotional during practice?

Completely normal. Breath and slow movement release accumulated tension. Pause, breathe, and continue when ready.

As you close this book, may you open a new chapter within yourself—
one where your breath guides you, your steps feel grounded,
and you trust your body's wisdom again.

These 28 days were never meant to be an ending.
They were a doorway back to presence, balance, and gentle strength.

And if you ever wonder why now, remember this truth: Nothing happens by accident.
And it is never too late to begin again. Whenever life feels heavy or uncertain, return to a movement, to a breath, to a moment of stillness.
Everything you need is already within you, quietly waiting.

Thank you for allowing me to walk beside you on this journey.
May your path ahead unfold with grace, softness, and a renewed sense of life. You are never walking alone.
You always have my support. I'm here—grateful, honored, and ready to accompany you whenever you choose to continue. Thank you for allowing me to walk beside you.

Thank you for allowing me to guide you towards your well-being, forever,

Fabiana Renacer

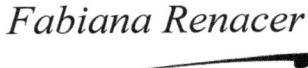

Before we part...

I want to thank you deeply for giving yourself this time and care.

Choosing to move gently, to listen to your body, and to honor your own rhythm is no small thing — especially at this stage of life.

If this book helped you feel calmer, more stable, more present in your body, or more confident in caring for yourself, your experience may be a meaningful gift to others who are looking for the same.

If you feel called to leave an honest review of this book, it would be truly appreciated.

You can do so on the same platform where you purchased the book.

Your voice may help someone else take their first gentle step.

And it's a great support that allows me to continue creating comprehensive and valuable programs for the well-being of older adults, thank you.

Here is the supplementary program for the book.
To access them, you may:

• **Scan the QR code included with this book.**

No video downloads are required.
Watch it instantly and practice anytime, on any device.

If you wish, you can have the PDF materials in print; they are enabled for one-click printing.

With gratitude,
Fabiana Renacer

Your bonuses are here 👆

www.ingramcontent.com/pod-product-compliance
Lightning Source LLC
Chambersburg PA
CBHW080524030426
42337CB00023B/4623